OTHER TITLES IN THIS SERIES

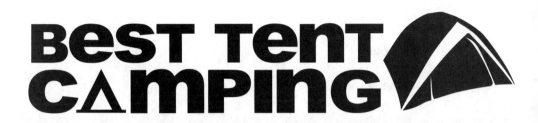

BEST TENT CAMPING
OHIO

YOUR CAR-CAMPING GUIDE TO SCENIC BEAUTY, THE SOUNDS OF NATURE, AND AN ESCAPE FROM CIVILIZATION

MENASHA RIDGE PRESS
BIRMINGHAM, ALABAMA

Best Tent Camping Ohio

Copyright © 2012 by Robert Loewendick

Printed in the United States of America
Published by Menasha Ridge Press
Distributed by Publishers Group West
First edition, first printing

Library of Congress Cataloging-in-Publication Data
   Loewendick, Robert.
      Best tent camping, Ohio : your car-camping guide to scenic beauty, the sounds of nature,
     and an escape from civilization / Robert Loewendick.
        p. cm.
     Includes index.
     ISBN-13: 978-0-89732-575-2
     ISBN-10: 0-89732-575-3
     1. Camp sites, facilities, etc.—Ohio—Guidebooks. 2. Camping—Ohio—Guidebooks.
     3. Ohio—Guidebooks. I. Title.
     GV191.42.O3L64 2012
     917.71068—dc23

                         2012008470

Cover design by Scott McGrew
Cover photo © joel zatz / Alamy
Text design by Ian Szymkowiak/Palace Press International, Inc.
Typesetting and composition by Annie Long
Cartography by Steve Jones and Robert Loewendick
Indexing by Rich Carlson

Menasha Ridge Press
P.O. Box 43673
Birmingham, Alabama 35243
www.menasharidge.com

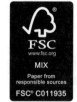
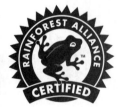

TABLE OF CONTENTS

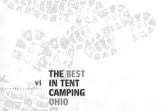

ACKNOWLEDGMENTS

ALTHOUGH ONE NAME IS PRINTED as the author on the cover, many people were involved in making this book a reality. I would like to give thanks to the people behind this book:

My acquisitions editor, Susan Haynes, for granting me the opportunity to research and write Ohio's great tent camping story. And to Holly Cross, the project editor, who guided me through this literary adventure.

Jean Backs and Sandy Chiaramonte with the ODNR Division of Parks for a steady stream of information when I requested it. And to the dedicated state park employees who keep Ohio's parks in order, even though they are restricted with funding issues.

The information officers of the metroparks, conservation districts, and national forests: Jeanne Dietrich, Paige Hosier, Darrin Lautenschleger, Tammy Ridout, and Gary Chancey.

To my four siblings, who at one point or another shared Ohio's outdoor wonders with me as a child and/or as an adult. Those adventures were always a big time for this tagalong and fuel for inspiring me to pursue outdoor/travel journalism.

To my parents, for providing nearly endless access to the outside, and with love and guidance.

To my wife, Linda, who patiently stoked the home fire while I was traveling around the state exploring campgrounds. And for sharing life's adventure hand in hand with me.

To my daughter, Danielle, and son, Rob, my most cherished gifts experienced while on this planet: They're great explorers in their own right and my best, lifelong camping buddies.

PREFACE

WHEN LOOKING OVER A LIST of the states that offer wilderness-type tent camping, Ohio wouldn't be in the lineup. But Ohio does hold some of the best tent camping in the country, in places that allow campers to rub elbows with an abundance of natural resources. I traveled around and through the state in search of those places that may have an edge over others—and I found them.

I conducted my campground reviews throughout one year, during Ohio's four seasons. Although I primarily focused my travel during the summer tent-camping season, usually when folks have a break from the annual grind of making a living, the spring and fall seasons were the most refreshing times for camping in the Buckeye State. Ohio's diverse landscape was and is a treat to see and experience, from wide rivers and great lakes, to quiet woodlots with natural bounties and heavily forested gorges as well. It was a pleasure to pitch the tent in these places and absorb the serenity they presented. I snapped thousands of photos and videos to assist in capturing the essence of the places that are revealed in the pages of this book.

While visiting many of these campgrounds, I met the dedicated staff and volunteers who massage the parks with loving hands and hearts. Those folks also shared with me their opinions of what made their park unique and how to experience it for myself—and for you. Most of my stays were just one-nighters, but with the scoop from the locals, I knew what to see and do. Some of the see-and-dos were in the campground, or near it; others were a short hike or paddle from camp; and some required a 5-mile drive or so. Wherever the adventure was, it was worth the trip.

During some of my travels, I was accompanied by my wife and two kids, and a portion of the research was with only my son. As we arrived at a park and began to see what it had to offer, I was mindful to observe the family's initial and departing reactions to the place. I noticed what caught their eyes and held their attention. I added those reactions to the research cooking pot as an ingredient to create a profile of the campground with an accurate viewpoint. I have revealed the highlights of each destination, but I also held back a few pleasant surprises that you will enjoy discovering on your own. Ohio has much to experience, so pack the tent and camp box and get started!

BORN AND RAISED IN OHIO, Robert still calls the Buckeye State his "base camp." Robert's decades of outdoor experiences are shared with others via writing and photography that have been published across North America. His diverse outdoor pursuits and travels continue to provide compelling stories and images that encourage others to get out there.

Spending days and nights surrounded by the natural world is not a hobby, but instead a lifestyle, for Robert. Whether fly-fishing a mountain stream or cruising a Great Lake for angling adventures, hiking miles of tame trails or wild ones, paddling calm waters or running rapids, Robert's days outdoors regularly end at a campsite. His dedication to promoting the wonders of the outdoors to others extends to his wife and two children, who frequently accompany him on his adventures and share stories around the evening campfire.

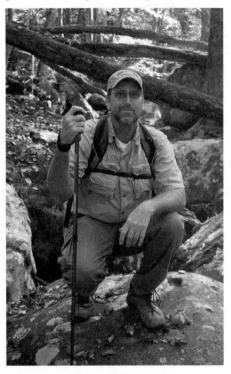

Robert is an active member of Outdoor Writers of Ohio and Outdoor Writers Association of America.

THE BEST OHIO CAMPGROUNDS

A Word about This Book and
Ohio Tent Camping

OHIO'S DIVERSITY OF RECREATIONAL OPPORTUNITIES is as varied as the state's geography. From fishing Lake Erie to hiking the Hocking Hills region, from paddling the Little Miami River north of Cincinnati to touring wineries of the northeast, Ohio is a legitimate travel destination. Exploring Ohio's treasures while tent camping puts the visitor in touch with a landscape and culture that appreciate life's simple pleasures.

The Muskingum Water Conservancy District manages several lakes in the east-central region that attract boaters and anglers. The state's largest state park, Salt Fork State Park, is a grand park for sure. Just about every outdoor activity you can think of happens there. The Wayne National Forest covers nearly half of the southeastern region. From driving roads that follow the Little Muskingum River to paddling tranquil lakes that rest in the valleys of the rugged hills, a picturesque camping experience can be found in this corner of Ohio. Primitive camping enthusiasts will appreciate American Electric Power's ReCreation Land—reclaimed coal mining lands that host more than 350 ponds and several campgrounds.

The hills meet the flatlands in the southwestern corner of the state. Slip into Shawnee State Park, nicknamed "The Little Smokies" for good reason. Great Seal and Scioto Trail state parks are in the heart of Native American lands, and several parks in the area present the Native American culture with burial mounds and museums.

Some of the most scenic camping in the state is on the Lake Erie Islands. South Bass Island features campsites with vistas overlooking the big lake. Reachable by ferry, the islands are a summer vacation destination. If the island campgrounds are full or mainland camping is your preference, East Harbor State Park campground will provide what you need.

For a nice blend of river, rugged hills, and primitive camping, the Mohican-Loudonville area between Cleveland and Columbus is the place. Clear Fork Gorge is a photographer's dream. Large hemlocks, rock outcroppings, and waterfalls are the backdrop to camping in this region.

So toss this book in the car and begin your tour of Ohio's natural destinations.

THE OVERVIEW MAP AND OVERVIEW-MAP KEY

Use the overview map on the inside front cover to determine the exact location of each campground. The campground's number appears not only on the overview map but also on the map key facing the overview map, in the table of contents, and on the profile's first page.

The book is organized by region, as indicated in the table of contents. A map legend that details the symbols found on the campground-layout maps appears on the inside back cover.

CAMPGROUND-LAYOUT MAPS

Each profile contains a detailed campground-layout map that provides an overhead view of campground sites, internal roads, facilities, and other key items.

GPS CAMPGROUND-ENTRANCE COORDINATES

Backpackers and campers were the first group to adopt GPS technology. Now it seems everyone has a box squawking directions on their dashboard. As GPS tools have become more and more affordable, it makes a lot of sense to include that information in each profile. This book gives each campground's location in latitude–longitude format.

THE CAMPGROUND PROFILE

In addition to maps, each profile contains a concise but informative narrative of the campground and individual sites. This descriptive text is enhanced with four helpful sidebars: Ratings, Key Information, Getting There (accurate driving directions that lead you to the campground from the nearest major roadway), and GPS Information. On the first page of each profile is a Ratings box.

THE RATING SYSTEM

For each campground, there's a rating from one to five for each of the following categories: beauty, privacy, spaciousness, quiet, security, and cleanliness. This was often a tough call because each section within each campground might warrant different ratings. So the ratings you'll see at the beginning of each profile are representative of the campground as a whole. While you may see a three or four for privacy overall, you can probably bet there are a couple of sites tucked in the far reaches of the campground that clearly rate a five.

BEAUTY This factor may seem obvious but is often elusive, or at the very least, subjective. What appeals to one camper may not appeal to another. All of the campgrounds in this guide are either in or near beautiful natural settings, and I've tried to describe those features in each profile. My rating for beauty focuses primarily on the campground itself.

PRIVACY When you set up your campsite, the last thing you want is to feel as if you're piled up on top of your neighbors. Even in campgrounds where the sites aren't huge, if they are encircled by a relatively dense forest and arranged with an eye toward privacy, you can find a site that puts you in your own slice of the woods.

SPACIOUSNESS Some of the campsites I've seen in Ohio are just barely big enough for your tent, a picnic table, and a fire ring. Others are large enough to accommodate a house. I don't typically need a lot of room when I'm camping, but I don't want to pitch my tent right next to the picnic table. This rating will give you an idea of how much elbow room you can expect when you set up camp.

QUIET Some parks tend to attract a rowdy crowd from Memorial Day through Labor Day. Groups of children running to and fro through the campsites and grown-ups playing music long into the night are not everyone's idea of camping. Other campgrounds are relatively peaceful throughout the season. (Keep in mind, however, that any public campground can attract a party crowd, especially on holiday weekends. Thankfully, this situation isn't as likely at the more remote locations.)

SECURITY The size of the campground and proximity to urban areas are the primary aspects I considered when making my security determinations. Be prudent, even when it looks like there's no one around. It's not a bad idea to lock up your car and your bike when you retire to your tent for the night. A little bit of precaution can go a long way toward making sure you return home with all your gear.

CLEANLINESS Each campground is rated on its overall cleanliness. Bathrooms and showers, camp stores, and other common areas are inspected and rated. It is also important that the sites themselves are clear of litter and the reminders of previous campers.

FIRST-AID KIT

A useful first-aid kit may contain more items than you might think necessary. These are just the basics. Prepackaged kits in waterproof bags (Atwater Carey and Adventure Medical make them) are available. As a preventive measure, take along sunscreen and insect repellent. Even though quite a few items are listed here, they pack down into a small space.

Ace bandages or Spenco joint wraps

Adhesive bandages, such as Band-Aids

Antibiotic ointment (Neosporin or the generic equivalent)

Antiseptic or disinfectant, such as Betadine or hydrogen peroxide

Aspirin or acetaminophen

Benadryl or the generic equivalent, diphenhydramine (in case of allergic reactions)

Butterfly-closure bandages

Comb and tweezers (for removing stray cactus needles from your skin)

Emergency poncho

Epinephrine in a prefilled syringe (for people known to have severe allergic reactions to such things as bee stings)

Gauze (one roll)

Gauze compress pads (six 4- x 4-inch pads)

LED flashlight or headlamp

Matches or pocket lighter

Mirror for signaling passing aircraft

Moleskin/Spenco "Second Skin"

Pocketknife or multipurpose tool

Waterproof first-aid tape

Whistle (it's more effective in signaling rescuers than your voice)

PLANNING YOUR OHIO CAMPING TRIP

The camping season in Ohio stretches from April to November at most campgrounds. Most Ohio State Parks are open year-round, but shower houses are closed and water supplies are turned off during winter. If you're geared up appropriately, spending a night in Ohio's winter landscape is refreshing. Winters can last a few months, so as soon as there is a hint of spring in the air, campers come out of their dens ready for some outdoor recreation. So, it's a good idea to make a reservation or have a plan B if you choose the first-come, first-serve method.

Many outdoor enthusiasts spend their summer vacations camping in Ohio, so you will find a few popular campsites occupied in the middle of the week. Ohio summers feel like Florida during July and August because of the high humidity that blankets the state, with temperatures in the 90s. Plan to pack a lot of ice to keep food safe and to create plenty of drinking water. Wooded sites are a premium, with campers looking for a cool campsite. When camping in the hill country, pick a site on a north-facing slope to drop the air temp at camp another couple degrees.

October brings out the leaf peepers, especially across the southern half of the state. Camping in Ohio during autumn is as good as tent camping gets: the aroma of falling leaves mixed with the smell of a campfire floating about the campground, cool nights for sleeping and warm days for relaxing or adventuring, and sights that demand multiple photos of each brightly colored scene.

Camping gear used for tent camping on a Lake Erie island is suitable for a camping trip to a deep-forest camp in the southern hill country. Although the campsites and surrounding regions are diverse in landscape, the camping method is identical. The basics are all that is needed. There are no wild critters to really be worried about, but bear sightings do occur along the eastern and southern border of the state. Ohio's country roads lead to some out-of-the-way places that are a pleasure to experience. The people of the Buckeye State are very hospitable and don't hesitate to offer a hand if you run into a problem on the road or at the campground.

Weather

Spring is the most variable season. During March, the hardwood trees begin to bud and the nights remain cool. Both winter- and summerlike weather can occur in spring. As summer approaches, the temperatures head for the 80s and often spike into the 90s. Summertime thunderstorms are brief but wild at times, with strong wind gusts. In fall, warm days and cool nights are the norm.

The first snows of winter usually arrive in December, and snow falls intermittently through March. About 40 to 120 inches of snow can fall during this time. Expect to incur entire days of below-freezing weather, though temperatures may range from mild to bitterly cold.

Helpful Hints

- An updated road map is a nice companion to bring along, as several roads have been abandoned and you may end up at a dead end. A GPS unit is a decent tool to back up the paper map, or vice versa.

- Ohio's gravel county and township roads are like driving on marbles during the summer road-grading season. Slow down and enjoy the view—and not from the ditch.

- The northern edge of Ohio is Lake Erie's shoreline. Storms come off the lake quickly and intensely throughout the spring and summer, so keep an eye on the horizon. Summer afternoon storms also form quickly and often release heavy downpours. When camping in the deep valleys of southern Ohio, consider this before leaving out for your camping trip. During the last decade, several Ohio campgrounds that lie at the bottom of sharp valleys have dealt with flash flooding.

- Wayne National Forest is split into three sections across southeastern Ohio. Although several destinations within the forest offer designated campsites, dispersed camping is also allowed. Camping is permitted on national forest lands anywhere that camping equipment or a vehicle does not block developed trails or right-of-ways. There is no charge for dispersed camping in the Wayne, but you must carry out any trash and abide the 14-day minimum stay law.

- The Ohio Department of Natural Resources' Department of Natural Areas and Preserves maintains 134 sites across the state. The natural areas are pristine places for visitors to get a look (don't touch!) at Ohio's true flora and fauna. Contact the DNAP for more information at (614) 265-6453.

- During the summer season and fall foliage season, it's best to reserve a campsite, if possible. Camping in Ohio during these seasons is busy, and securing a campsite can be a challenge. For first-come, first-serve sites, call ahead to the campground office to find out if those sites are still available. If you choose not to call ahead, showing up on Friday as early as possible will increase your odds of grabbing a site.

Roads and Vehicles

While doing the research for this book and bumping along dirt roads all over the state, we reset our standards for what constitutes a good road. We consider a good road to be well-graded gravel, wide, with few rocks or dips, where we can clip along at 30 mph. The majority of these campgrounds can be reached by a careful driver in a standard sedan when the roads are dry. For the most part, Ohio's roads are paved. The gravel roads and campground lanes don't require a four-wheel drive vehicle. Obey all traffic signs and keep in mind that vehicles driving uphill have the right-of-way on narrow roads.

Get a good, detailed map, like the DeLorme Gazetteer, if you intend to travel the back roads, make sure your vehicle's in good shape, and carry an emergency kit with plenty of water.

Permits and Access

All of Ohio's state parks are accessible without a permit. The metroparks may charge a small fee for entry, which is payable at the park entrance. The AEP ReCreation Land requires a user permit to camp, fish, or simply explore. To get a free permit, visit AEP's website at **www.aep.com/environmental/recreation/recland/permit.aspx** or one of the regional sporting goods stores or bait shops surrounding the recreational lands.

ANIMAL AND PLANT HAZARDS

Snakes

Ohio has a variety of snakes—including garter, black rat, and racers—most of which are benign. Timber rattlesnakes are occasionally spotted along the forested hills in extreme southern Ohio. Copperheads are more common across the southern half of the state and can be fairly aggressive if agitated.

When hiking, stick to well-used trails and wear over-the-ankle boots and loose-fitting long pants. Rattlesnakes like to bask in the sun and won't bite unless threatened. Do not step or put your hands where you cannot see and avoid wandering around in the dark. Step on logs and rocks, never over them, and be especially careful when climbing rocks or gathering firewood.

Ticks

Ticks are often found on brush and tall grass, waiting to hitch a ride on a warm-blooded passerby. They are most active during the summer months. You can use several strategies to reduce your chances of ticks getting under your skin. Some people choose to wear light-colored clothing, so ticks can be spotted before they make it to the skin. Most important, be sure to visually check your hair, back of neck, armpits, and socks at the end of the hike. During your posthike shower, take a moment to do a more complete body check. For ticks that are already embedded, removal with tweezers is best. Use disinfectant solution on the wound.

Poison Ivy

Poison Ivy is a common plant growing throughout Ohio. These itch-causing plants do grow near perennial streams and ponds. Recognizing and avoiding poison ivy is the most effective way to prevent the painful, itchy rashes associated with these plants. Poison ivy occurs as a vine or groundcover, 3 leaflets to a leaf. Urushiol, the oil in the sap of poison ivy, is responsible for the rash. Within 14 hours of exposure, raised lines and/or blisters will appear on the affected area, accompanied by a terrible itch. Refrain from scratching because bacteria under your fingernails can cause an infection. Wash and dry the rash thoroughly, applying a calamine lotion to help dry out the rash. If itching or blistering is severe, seek medical attention. If you do come into contact with one of these plants, remember that oil-contaminated clothes, pets, or hiking gear can easily cause an irritating rash on you or someone else, so wash not only any exposed parts of your body but also clothes, gear, and pets, if applicable.

TIPS FOR A HAPPY CAMPING TRIP

There is nothing worse than a bad camping trip, especially because it is so easy to have a great time. To assist with making your outing a happy one, here are some pointers.

- **RESERVE YOUR SITE AHEAD OF TIME,** especially if it's a weekend, a holiday, or if the campground is wildly popular. Many prime campgrounds require at least a six-month lead time on reservations. Check before you go.

- **PICK YOUR CAMPING BUDDIES WISELY.** A family trip is pretty straightforward, but you may want to reconsider including grumpy Uncle Fred, who doesn't like bugs, sunshine, or marshmallows. After you know who's going, make sure that everyone is on the same page regarding expectations of difficulty (amenities or the lack thereof, physical exertion, and so on), sleeping arrangements, and food requirements.

- **DON'T DUPLICATE EQUIPMENT,** such as cooking pots and lanterns, among campers in your party. Carry what you need to have a good time, but don't turn the trip into a major moving experience.

- **DRESS FOR THE SEASON.** Educate yourself on the temperature highs and lows of the specific area you plan to visit. It may be warm at night in the summer in your backyard, but up in the mountains it will be quite chilly.

- **PITCH YOUR TENT ON A LEVEL SURFACE,** preferably one covered with leaves, pine straw, or grass. Use a tarp or specially designed footprint to thwart ground moisture and to protect the tent floor. Do a little site maintenance, such as picking up the small rocks and sticks that can damage your tent floor and make sleep uncomfortable. If you have a separate tent rain fly but don't think you'll need it, keep it rolled up at the base of the tent in case it starts raining at midnight.

- **IF YOU ARE NOT COMFORTABLE SLEEPING ON THE GROUND,** take a sleeping pad with you that is full-length and thicker than you think you might need. This will not only keep your hips from aching on hard ground but will also help keep you warm. A wide range of thin, light, inflatable pads is available at camping stores today, and these are a much better choice than home air mattresses, which conduct heat away from the body and tend to deflate during the night.

- **IF YOU'RE NOT HIKING IN TO A PRIMITIVE CAMPSITE,** there is no real need to skimp on food due to weight. Plan tasty meals and bring everything you will need to prepare, cook, eat, and clean up.

- **IF YOU TEND TO USE THE BATHROOM MULTIPLE TIMES AT NIGHT,** you should plan ahead. Leaving a warm sleeping bag and stumbling around in the dark to find the restroom, whether it be a pit toilet, a fully plumbed comfort station, or just the woods, is not fun. Keep a flashlight and any other accoutrements you may need by the tent door and know exactly where to head in the dark.

- **STANDING DEAD TREES AND STORM-DAMAGED LIVING TREES** can pose a real hazard to tent campers. These trees may have loose or broken limbs that could fall at any time. When choosing a campsite, or even just a spot to rest during a hike, look up.

CAMPING ETIQUETTE

Camping experiences can vary wildly, depending on a variety of factors, such as weather, preparedness, fellow campers, and time of year. Here are a few tips on how to create good vibes with fellow campers and wildlife you encounter.

- **OBTAIN ALL PERMITS AND AUTHORIZATION AS REQUIRED.** Be sure you check in, pay your fee, and mark your site as directed. Don't make the mistake of grabbing a seemingly empty site that is more appealing than your site. It could be reserved. If you're unhappy with your site, check with the campground host for other options.

- **LEAVE ONLY FOOTPRINTS.** Be sensitive to the ground beneath you. Be sure to place all garbage in designated receptacles or pack it out if none is available. No one likes to see the trash someone else has left behind.

- **NEVER SPOOK ANIMALS.** It's common for animals to wander through campsites, where they may be accustomed to the presence of humans (and our food). An unannounced approach, a sudden movement, or a loud noise startles most animals. A surprised animal can be dangerous to you, to others, and to themselves. Give them plenty of space.

- **PLAN AHEAD.** Know your equipment, your ability, and your camping area—and prepare accordingly. Be self-sufficient at all times; carry necessary supplies for changes in weather or other conditions. A well-executed trip is a satisfaction to you and to others.

- **BE COURTEOUS TO CAMPERS, HIKERS, BIKERS, AND OTHERS YOU ENCOUNTER.** If you run into the owner of a large RV, don't panic. Just wave, feign eye contact, and then walk slowly away.

- **STRICTLY FOLLOW THE CAMPGROUND'S RULES REGARDING THE BUILDING OF FIRES.** Never burn trash. Trash smoke smells horrible, and trash debris in a fire pit or grill is unsightly.

Campground Courtesy

This stuff is common sense, but like a lot of common sense, it bears repeating. Be aware of the quiet hours, especially when pulling into a campground after dark. Avoid shining your headlights or flashlights into other campsites as you are searching for a spot. And please turn down your car stereo; that bass beat carries very well in the night. Always walk on the designated paths and roads and respect the privacy of your neighbors by not strolling through their sites to get to the restrooms. You'll also reduce damage to the foliage and keep the campground green by sticking to the main trail. Please clean up after yourself. Make cleaning up into a game with your kids: Whoever packs out the most twist-ties, pop tops, and gum wrappers is the winner.

BACKCOUNTRY-CAMPING ADVICE

A permit is not required before entering the backcountry to camp in the Wayne National Forest. However, you should practice low-impact camping. Adhere to the adages "Pack it in, pack it out" and "Take only pictures, leave only footprints." Practice leave-no-trace camping ethics while in the backcountry.

Open fires are permitted except during dry times when the forest service may issue a fire ban. Backpacking stoves are strongly encouraged.

Solid human waste should be buried in a hole at least three inches deep and at least 200 feet away from trails and water sources; a trowel is basic backpacking equipment. More and more often, however, the practice of burying human waste is being banned. Using a portable latrine (it comes in various incarnations and is basically a glorified plastic bag) may seem unthinkable at first, but it's really no big deal. Just bring an extra large zip-top bag for extra insurance against structural failures.

Following the above guidelines will increase your chances for a pleasant, safe, and low-impact interaction with nature.

VENTURING AWAY FROM THE CAMPGROUND

If you go for a hike, bike, or other excursion into the wilderness, here are some tips.

- **ALWAYS CARRY FOOD AND WATER,** whether you are planning to go overnight or not. Food will give you energy, help keep you warm, and sustain you in an emergency until help arrives. Bring potable water or treat water by boiling or filtering before drinking from a lake or stream.

- **STAY ON DESIGNATED TRAILS.** Most hikers get lost when they leave the trail. Even on the most clearly marked trails, there is usually a point where you have to stop and consider which direction to head. If you become disoriented, don't panic. As soon as you think you may be off-track, stop, assess your current direction, and then retrace your steps back to the point where you went awry. If you have absolutely no idea how to continue, return to the trailhead the way you came in. Should you become completely lost and have no idea of how to return to the trailhead, remaining in place along the trail and waiting for help is most often the best option for adults and always the best option for children.

- **BE ESPECIALLY CAREFUL WHEN CROSSING STREAMS.** Whether you are fording the stream or crossing on a log, make every step count. If you have any doubt about maintaining your balance on a log, go ahead and ford the stream instead. When fording a stream, use a trekking pole or stout stick for balance and face upstream as you cross. If a stream seems too deep to ford, turn back. Whatever is on the other side is not worth risking your life.

- **BE CAREFUL AT OVERLOOKS.** Although these areas may provide spectacular views, they are potentially hazardous. Stay back from the edge of outcrops and be absolutely sure of your footing: A misstep can mean a nasty and possibly fatal fall.

- **KNOW THE SYMPTOMS OF HYPOTHERMIA.** Shivering and forgetfulness are the two most common indicators of this insidious killer. Hypothermia can occur at any elevation, even in the summer. Wearing cotton clothing puts you especially at risk because cotton, when wet, wicks heat away from the body. To prevent hypothermia, dress in layers using synthetic clothing for insulation, use a cap and gloves to reduce heat loss, and protect yourself with waterproof, breathable outerwear. If symptoms arise, get the victim to shelter and a fire, into dry clothes or a dry sleeping bag, and administer hot liquids.

- **TAKE ALONG YOUR BRAIN.** A cool, calculating mind is the single most important piece of equipment you'll ever need on the trail. Think before you act. Watch your step. Plan ahead. Avoiding accidents before they happen is the best recipe for a rewarding and relaxing hike.

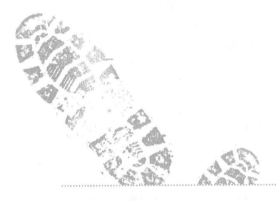

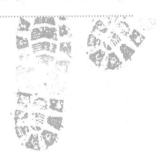

NORTHWEST

1
KISER LAKE STATE PARK

THIS QUIET, SMALLER PARK (531 acres) offers big benefits to the camper wanting to get away. Surrounded by wooded hills and diverse wetlands, Kiser State Park is a wildlife viewers' goldmine. This diverse landscape was created by glaciers that left deposits of boulders, sand, and gravel. Many of the boulders and sands were gathered by the glaciers as they headed south from Canada. The rock found lying around the short hills and washes surrounding the lake date from the glacial period. This area was also the home of Tecumseh, the great Shawnee warrior. Hiking the 11 miles of park trails reveals the natural amenities that supported the area's Native Americans. For anglers, there are five stone fishing piers placed around the lake near various forms of game fish habitat. Kiser Lake is off limits to boats with engines, so feel free to paddle away without any wake to contend with while trying to get that close-up water photo.

A diverse campground starts at the lake's southern shoreline and extends up into the woods. Arriving from the south, the campground entrance is on the right after passing a stately row of weeping willows. The lake is also on the left, and 14 sites are sprinkled along its shore, about the 50-yard distance from the road to the lake. Back to the main section of the campground you will find sites 30–51 in orderly rows, in full sun. Slide through that group and find site 29 as the campground lane curves along the southern edge and heads toward a wood grove. Sites 23–28 are on the right as you approach the wood grove, and while a bit small and close to the road, they are comfortable sites with a woodland backing.

Sites 12–22 line both sides of the 200-foot paved lane leading through the center of the wood grove. Sites 21 and 22 are nonreservable (titled "walk-in sites" in the Ohio State Parks system). Sites 15 and 16 sit at the cul de sac at the head of the wood grove and are great tent

> *The glaciers shaped Kiser's diverse landscapes of wetlands, forest, and lake.*

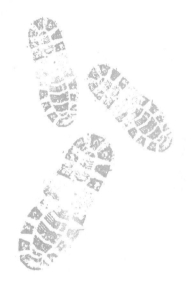

RATINGS

Beauty: ✩ ✩ ✩
Privacy: ✩ ✩
Spaciousness: ✩ ✩
Quiet: ✩ ✩ ✩
Security: ✩ ✩ ✩
Cleanliness: ✩ ✩ ✩

ADDRESS: 4889 North State Route 235 Conover, OH 45317

OPERATED BY: ODNR Division of State Parks

INFORMATION: (937) 362-3565; www.dnr.state. oh.us/parks

RESERVATIONS: (866) 644-6727; www.ohio.reserve world.com

OPEN: Year-round; limited facilities in winter months

SITES: 108 nonelectric; 10 electric

EACH SITE: Picnic table, fire ring

ASSIGNMENT: Reservable sites; nonelectric sites first come, first served

REGISTRATION: Self-registration station at campground entrance

FACILITIES: Pit latrines, camp store, boat rental, sports courts, playground, swimming beach

PARKING: At each site

FEE: $23 electric; $19 nonelectric

ELEVATION: 1,108 feet

RESTRICTIONS: *Pets:* On leash only *Fires:* In fire ring *Alcohol:* Prohibited *Vehicles:* 2 per site *Other:* Quiet hours 10 p.m.–8 a.m.; gathering firewood prohibited; limit 6 persons per site

sites, as they do require a short walk (ten yards) in. The Red Oak hiking trail passes by site 18 and connects with the Boardwalk Trail to the west.

The Boardwalk Trail guides visitors through the Kiser Lake Wetlands—a 51-acre State Nature Preserve. The boardwalk is also accessible from a small parking area 0.2 mile south of the campground entrance. The wetlands include two prairie fens that are home to numerous rare plant species, animals, and insects. The Giant Swallowtail butterfly and the Northern Ravine salamander are two residents you may see while walking along the 0.6-mile, looping boardwalk.

Across the road from the main campground are those waterfront sites. Sites 66–71 sit directly across from the main campground entrance, spread around a small, paved circle. Site 71 is the closest to the water, but it also is heavily visited by Canada Geese, which leave behind unpleasant droppings. Sites 72–75 are across a drainage ditch to the north and accessible from their own paved road. Each of these sites has a shade tree and a wide view of the lake. Just to the north of those four sites is the last quad of sites, sites 76–79, also separated from the prior by a drainage ditch. Site 79 is the only one in this group with shade and sits on the water's edge. During midsummer, expect mats of lily pads to be parked along the shoreline, which make it tough to fish from the campsite.

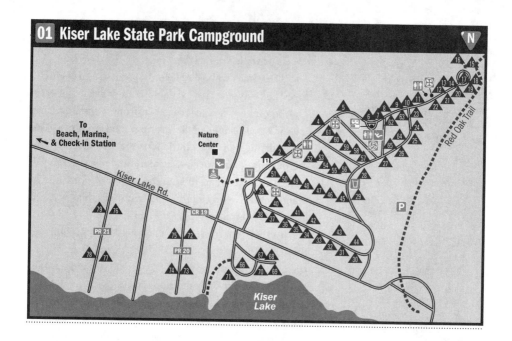

01 Kiser Lake State Park Campground

To Beach, Marina, & Check-in Station

Nature Center

Kiser Lake Rd.

CR 19

PR 21

PR 20

Red Oak Trail

Kiser Lake

GETTING THERE

From Piqua, at I-75 Exit 82, travel east on US 36 for 12.18 miles to OH 235 on the left. Follow OH 235 north for 3.01 miles to Possum Run Road on the right. Go 1.51 miles to Kiser Lake Road, turn left, and follow for 0.89 mile to the campground entrance on the right.

GPS COORDINATES

N40°10.979'
W83°56.934'

2
LAKE LORAMIE STATE PARK

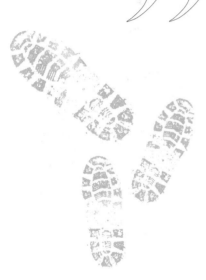

This lake, built in 1824, fed the Miami–Erie Canal system, which is traced by hiking trails today.

LAKE **L**ORAMIE **S**TATE **P**ARK is built around the remnants of the Miami–Erie Canal. The lake was constructed in 1824 to store water to supply the canal system that provided transportation between Lake Erie and the Ohio River. A section of the park's trail system follows the Miami–Erie Canal, which is also a part of the Buckeye Trail and the North Country National Scenic Trail. Plenty of historical sites are nearby, as are artisans displaying their skills during spring, summer, and fall at a local art center neighboring the park. An assembly of bald cypress trees and sweet gum trees dating back to the 1950s are grown in the campground. Campers *must* pull out their fishing gear while at this park—easy shore fishing abounds around Lake Loramie. Picnic tables are also liberally dispersed around the many lagoons on the lake's west side.

West central Ohio isn't one of the state regions frequented by campers, but Lake Loramie State Park is an exception. The majority of the campground is frequented by RVers, and the flat park seems like a busy neighborhood of little white homes during the summer vacation season. The exception, however, are the nonelectric sites that sit alone on a square peninsula, somewhat separated from the RV village. There are two sets of sites sharing the same numbers, 1–14. The first 14-site section is electric and is located a couple yards north of the campground office at the campground entrance—ignore those. Instead, take a right after passing by the campground office by site 135 on the right. Then take a left before site 152, then an immediate right, and cruise by sites 92–95. Next to site 95 is signage on the left directing you to the overflow parking access road—follow that. The peninsula, approximately 50 yards by 50 yards, is on the right. Dressed with a few massive oak trees standing in the middle are the nonelectric sites 1–14. This is where you want to be, but be aware that these sites are not reservable.

RATINGS

Beauty: ✩ ✩
Privacy: ✩ ✩
Spaciousness: ✩ ✩ ✩
Quiet: ✩ ✩ ✩
Security: ✩ ✩ ✩ ✩
Cleanliness: ✩ ✩ ✩ ✩

The nonelectric section is not completely cut off from the two main camping areas, and the RVs are not completely out of sight, but the nonelectric sites focus on the lake channel that surrounds the peninsula. The channel, or canal, of Lake Loramie is nearly at ground level, so sliding a kayak into the water from the campsite is doable. Paddle the channel under the footbridge and out into bigger water if you dare.

The nonelectric sites are split into two sections. The first sites as you arrive on the peninsula are sites 1–4. There is only a hint of a path for your vehicle to follow to the sites from the gravel lane, but it's legal to drive on the grass at that point. These first four sites are at the water's edge, as are sites 5 and 6. Sites 7–9 are on the interior of the peninsula, completing a horseshoe shape that is one of the two sections. The second subsection of the nonelectric peninsula has sites 10–14, which sit at the water's edge along the peninsula's eastern shore. Parking for those five sites is on the graveled loop that starts behind site 9 and ends at the front of site 14. These five sites are prime because they face the canal laced with American lotus and the opposing bank covered with vegetation that supports migrating waterfowl. A shower house and water supply are back by site 152.

A footbridge crossing the lake channel near site 14 leads to the 2-mile Lakeview Trail. This is an easy walk, level except for the bridge crossing. Another footbridge leading to the island sits at the trail's turning point, at the Blackberry Island Access parking area. A nature trail follows the forested island's perimeter and puts you one-on-one with the busy birds that live at and visit the island.

Note: Persons under 18 years old must have written consent of a parent or legal guardian to register for a campsite.

KEY INFORMATION

ADDRESS: 4401 Ft. Loramie Swanders Road Minster, OH 45865

OPERATED BY: ODNR Division of State Parks

INFORMATION: (937) 295-2011; www.dnr.state.oh.us/parks

RESERVATIONS: (866) 644-6727; www.ohio.reserveworld.com

OPEN: Year-round; limited facilities in winter; showers closed November–March

SITES: 15 nonelectric; 160 electric

EACH SITE: Picnic table, fire ring

ASSIGNMENT: Reservable sites; walk-in sites first come, first served

REGISTRATION: Self-registration station at campground office, if office closed

FACILITIES: Showers, flush toilets, laundry, camp store, sports courts, playground, swimming beach, miniature golf, nature center

PARKING: At each site

FEE: $21 nonelectric; $25 electric

ELEVATION: 950 feet

RESTRICTIONS: *Pets:* On leash only *Fires:* In fire ring *Alcohol:* Prohibited *Vehicles:* 2 per site *Other:* Quiet hours 10 p.m.–8 a.m.; gathering firewood prohibited; limit 6 persons per site

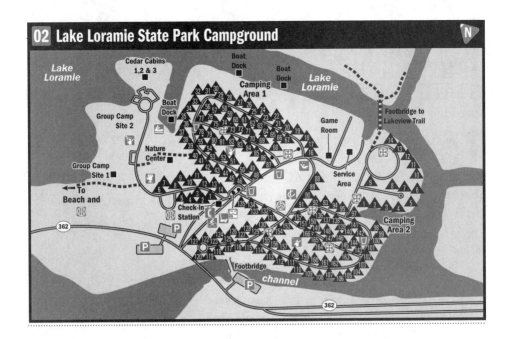

GETTING THERE

From I-75 Exit 99 near Anna, go west on OH 119 for 10.6 miles to Minster. Turn left on South Paris Street at the outskirts of town, follow to OH 362 and turn left. Follow OH 362 for 2.51 miles to the campground entrance on the left.

GPS COORDINATES

N40°21.459'
W84°21.430'

3
MARY JANE THURSTON STATE PARK

THE MAUMEE RIVER, a State Scenic River, has been a vital passageway for centuries and then some. Native Americans utilized the river for sustenance and travel—two elements still experienced there today, on a recreational level. The Mary Jane Thurston State Park provides access to the river and its supporting environment, especially on the southern riverbank west of Grand Rapids. Grand Rapids itself is a neat little river town that caters to river visitors with shops, ice-cream parlors, and a great view of the river and its historic canal system. A day-use area and campground lie just west of Grand Rapids. The day-use area includes a small lodge overlooking the river and an observation deck. Keep your eye to the sky, as bald eagles are regularly spotted here searching for a meal. Across the river, northwest of the campground and day-use area, is the North Turkeyfoot area of the state park. To get there, leave the campground entrance and travel 7.37 miles west on OH 65 to a bridge; after crossing the bridge, turn right. On the right is the riverfront forest with various hiking trails that lead through heavy river woodlands habitat. Dispersed tent camping is allowed throughout North Turkeyfoot, but no fires are allowed.

Back at the campground, time can fly while sitting along the river's edge and pondering what it must have been like there a century ago. The campground consists of 35 sites separated into two sections. Near the campground entrance are the first 14 sites, considered RV sites. Sites 1–4 are equipped with water hookups but no electricity. The campground host occupies site 2 and sells firewood through the late spring, summer, and early fall camping seasons. A footbridge at the back side of site 2 leads to the park's day-use area. Sites 5–14 are on the left side of the campground road, opposite the first four. The sites are staged along both sides of a spur road that leads to a small parking area and the base

> *Explore the historic Maumee River while camping riverside.*

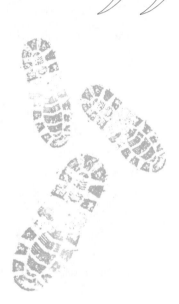

RATINGS

Beauty: ✩ ✩ ✩
Privacy: ✩ ✩
Spaciousness: ✩ ✩ ✩
Quiet: ✩ ✩
Security: ✩ ✩
Cleanliness: ✩ ✩

ADDRESS:	1466 State Route 65 McClure, OH 43534
OPERATED BY:	ODNR Division of State Parks
INFORMATION:	(419) 832-7662; www.dnr.state. oh.us/parks
RESERVATIONS:	(866) 644-6727; www.ohio.reserve world.com
OPEN:	Year-round but no water
SITES:	35 nonelectric
EACH SITE:	Picnic table, fire ring
ASSIGNMENT:	Reservable sites; walk-in sites first come, first served
REGISTRATION:	Self-registration station at camp- ground entrance
FACILITIES:	Portable toilets at tent area lot, water spigot and shower fixture mounted to rear of bulletin board at tent area lot, flush toilets at day-use lodge, marina and boat ramp, playground
PARKING:	At each site; in parking area for tent-only sites
FEE:	$19 nonelectric; $21 premium non- electric
ELEVATION:	639 feet
RESTRICTIONS:	*Pets:* On leash only *Fires:* In fire ring *Alcohol:* Prohibited *Vehicles:* 2 per site; no vehicles al- lowed in tent area *Other:* Quiet hours 10 p.m.–8 a.m.; gathering firewood prohibited; limit 6 persons per site

of the sledding hill. These spacious sites offer plenty of room for a boat trailer and a tent to fit comfortably.

Follow the gravel lane from the RV area through a woodlot toward the Maumee River. As the river comes into view, sites 15 and 16 will be on the right, next to the playground. These sites fill a corner created by the river and a feeder creek to the east. Because these sites are the first to greet visitors, they experience several daytime drive-bys by sightseers. The same goes for sites 16 and 17, around the corner and parallel to the river, which are neighbors to the two rental cabins. A small amphitheater sits between the last cabin and the small gravel parking lot designated for the tent camping area at the river's edge going west.

Sites 21–35 are strung out in two equal rows running along the river, only a few feet above the water. During early spring rains, the campground may be closed due to flooding, so call ahead to confirm that it is dry. During times of normal river levels, waders are common in the short, shallow falls within sight of the campground. Site 21 is the first site closest to the river from the parking lot. Site 35 is across the flat, grassy campground lawn, with a forested marsh at its back side. Site 29 is the farthest from the parking area, requiring a walk of 40 yards. Site 28 offers a wide, unobstructed view of the river and the falls. A hundred yards downstream are two dams, one on each side of a small island. The dams slow and deep-en the water at that point, making it a turning point for boaters and water skiers, who are entertaining to watch while enjoying a shoreside lunch at the campsite.

Site 27's river view is blocked by a short row of young trees, so, if a privacy screen from the river is de-sired, this is the site for you. Site 22 blends with the river's edge for easy access to fishing or cooling toes in the water working its way to Lake Erie, only 25 miles away. The Maumee River becomes crowded with wall-eye anglers during the spring spawning runs that begin when water temperatures reach just above freezing. The main attraction here is the river, so take advantage of the numerous ways to interact with it, whatever the season.

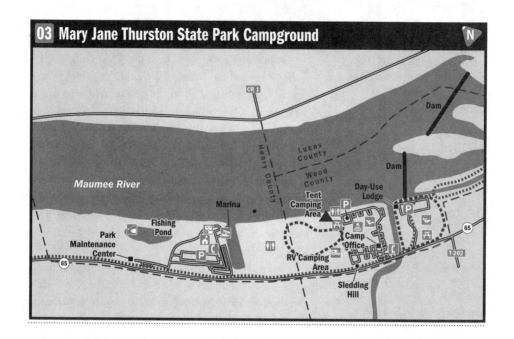

GETTING THERE

From I-75 Exit 179 at Bowling Green, take OH 6 west for 13.35 miles to CR 189 (Wapakoneta Road) on the right. Follow CR 189 north for 2.77 miles to OH 65 (W. 2nd Street) and turn left. Travel 0.71 mile to the campground entrance on the right.

GPS COORDINATES

N41°24.575'
W83°52.658'

4
WOLF CREEK PARK

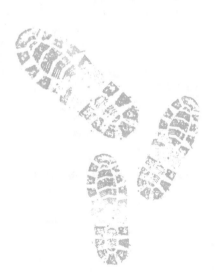

> *This quiet campground sits on the bank of a State Scenic River.*

THIS PARK GOT ITS NAME from the creek north of the park that is a tributary to the Sandusky River—a State Scenic River. The river received its scenic status in the early 1970s, the second river in Ohio to be tagged such. The 130-mile-long Sandusky River is a diverse watercourse that flows over stone falls at some points, and then slowly courses along stretches of deeper pools and runs. Time flies while paddling the river and taking in picturesque views of the riverscapes. A day on the river also brings on an appetite for tasty camp cooking and an outing iced with a night under the open, northern Ohio sky. Wolf Creek Park provides just the right situation for that adventure.

Two nature trails explore the river environment from the water's edge and then away from the water through fields of wildflowers during the spring and summer camping seasons. Check with park management for the dates conservationists will be conducting Stream Quality Monitoring at the canoe launch point at the picnic area, north of the campground. Samples of aquatic insects and other interesting things will be picked and plucked from under and between the river rocks. But don't be disappointed if you can't attend an organized exploration day on the river; simply slip on some old tennis shoes, grab a small net, wade on in, and see what you can find.

Although the campground runs along the western bank of the Sandusky River, the sites are not at the water's edge. Access to the river from even the closest campsite requires a 20-yard walk through knee-high vegetation and trees growing on a steep bank. But once you arrive at the water, the view and water are a pleasant reward. On quiet nights, you can still hear the river even with the tree and brush buffer between your site and the river. The first eight sites, beginning at the registration bulletin board, border both sides of the gravel

RATINGS

Beauty: ☆ ☆
Privacy: ☆ ☆ ☆
Spaciousness: ☆ ☆ ☆
Quiet: ☆ ☆ ☆
Security: ☆ ☆
Cleanliness: ☆ ☆ ☆

campground road. These sites are the smallest of the 24 sites. Next to site 15 is a well water supply pump only a couple yards off of the road. You may meet a backpacker or two at the pump, as the Buckeye Trail passes through the park.

The campground road passes through a pinch point with a wooded wash on both sides of the road. During times of high water, this wash may see some water, but there's no need to worry, as the elevation between the campground and the wash is more than 20 feet. The next three sites between the road and the river are the closest to the waterway. Each site has a footpath leading to the river, so a quick cast or two with the fly rod can be had before that simmering meal in the Dutch oven is ready to eat. Sites 16, 17, and 18 are on the river side as the campground road enters a 50-yard circle opening, while the remainder of the sites sit around the outer edge of the big loop surrounding a mowed lawn (good for chasing balls or flying a kite). The summer weekend I visited the park, ours was one of only two sites occupied. The campground is quiet except for OH 53, which can be a busy road during the day. The sites are well spread out with at least a dozen or so yards between them. Site 21 has a nature trail that passes through it; the trail then leads to the picnic area to the north of the campground and then turns south back to the registration bulletin board, where it connects to another nameless nature trail.

From the campground entrance off OH 53, travel north 0.91 mile up the highway to the picnic area and canoe launch access road. The canoe launch ramp is on the right at the end of a small gravel parking lot. Canoes and kayaks must be carried 75 feet down a paved decline to the river's edge. Across from the ramp is a small island splitting the river. For a 2-mile float down the Sandusky River, put in at the County Road 201 bridge north of the park and take out at the park's canoe launch ramp or at the gravel bank at the campground. The river is the reason for visiting Wolf Creek Park. No matter what level of interaction you prefer with this scenic river, it's worth your time.

KEY INFORMATION

ADDRESS: 2701 OH 53 Freemont, OH 43420

OPERATED BY: Sandusky County Park District

INFORMATION: (419) 334-4495; (888) 200-5577; www.lovemyparks. com/parks/wolf_ creek_park

RESERVATIONS: First come, first served

OPEN: April 1–December 31

SITES: 24 primitive

EACH SITE: Picnic table, fire ring

ASSIGNMENT: First come, first served

REGISTRATION: Self-registration at bulletin board on right at campground entrance

FACILITIES: Well water pumps, pit latrines, canoe launch ramp

PARKING: At each site

FEE: $15

ELEVATION: 667 feet

RESTRICTIONS: *Pets:* Must be leashed; do not tether to a tree *Fires:* In fire ring *Alcohol:* Prohibited *Vehicles:* 2 per site *Other:* Quiet hours 11 p.m.–7 a.m.; no firewood gathering; camping in designated areas only

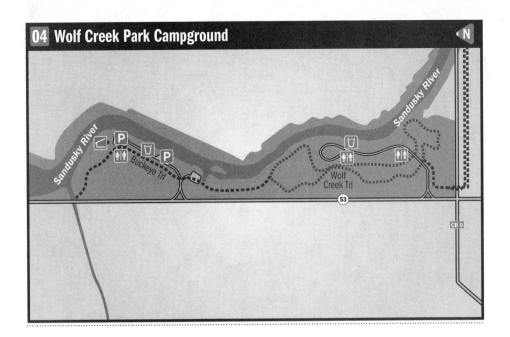

GETTING THERE

From Freemont, follow OH
53 south for 5.43 miles to
campground entrance on
the left.

GPS COORDINATES

N41°15.839'
W83°10.100'

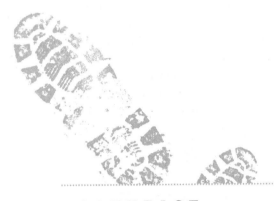

NORTHEAST

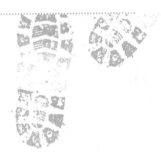

5
BEAVER CREEK STATE PARK

ARRIVING FROM THE NORTH, it's soon apparent to visitors that they have arrived at the doorstep to the Appalachian Mountains. Beaver Creek State Park covers 2,722 land acres and only 4 miles of river, but the river is the main attraction. The river has been designated a National Wild and Scenic River, and rightly so. Slip a kayak into the clear waters of Little Beaver Creek and shoot over a few short rapids for some whitewater fun, or simply lean back and admire the cliffs that contain the river. At the center of the park is a pioneer village that relied on the river to turn millstones during the early 1800s. An iron bridge crosses the river at the village, which is also the site of the park office. South of the village, 0.87 mile on Echo Dell Road, is the park's Wildlife Education Center (open weekends) that features live animals and 300 mounted specimens.

The family campground of Beaver Creek State Park offers tent campers the picture-perfect place to stake their nylon cabins. As soon as you pull into the campground, your mind will instantly transition from daily stress to relax-and-relent mode. Site 42 is the first site on the left. It sits only a dozen yards beyond the entrance, but its appearance and layout resembles a campsite in a western forest, with big pines spaced enough to give a non-confined sensation and a plush carpet of pine needles underfoot. After passing site 42, a road to the left leads to the best sites of the campground–sites 43–55. Sites 43, 44, and 45 are not reservable but honor a first-come, first-served status. The remaining sites are reservable.

This shorter road of the campground has campsites on the upper side only. Site 44 is several feet wider and deeper than the others, with white pines towering like giant soldiers. Site 46 lies in a slight swale that dips through the pine-covered ridge. Avoid this site if rain is in the weather forecast. This campground road goes for one-tenth of a mile before ending at a cul-de-sac. Near

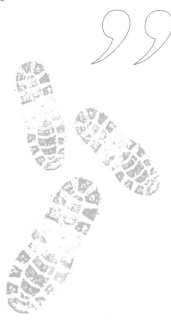

Little Beaver Creek, a National Wild and Scenic River, cuts through this forest wilderness.

RATINGS

Beauty: ☆ ☆ ☆ ☆
Privacy: ☆ ☆ ☆
Spaciousness: ☆ ☆ ☆
Quiet: ☆ ☆ ☆
Security: ☆ ☆ ☆
Cleanliness: ☆ ☆ ☆

KEY INFORMATION

ADDRESS: 12021 Echo Dell Rd.
East Liverpool,
OH 43920

OPERATED BY: ODNR Division of
State Parks

INFORMATION: (330) 385-309;
www.dnr.state
.oh.us/parks

RESERVATIONS: (866) 644-6727;
www.ohio
.reserveworld.com

OPEN: Year-round;
limited facilities
in winter

SITES: 44 nonelectric;
6 electric

EACH SITE: Picnic table, fire
ring

ASSIGNMENT: Reservable sites;
walk-in sites first
come, first served

REGISTRATION: Self-registration
station at camp-
ground

FACILITIES: Latrines, sun shower, playground,
nature center,
pioneer village

PARKING: At each site

FEE: $19; deduct $1
from fee Sunday–
Thursday; deduct
$2 in winter

ELEVATION: 1,102 feet

RESTRICTIONS: *Pets:* Allowed, but
must be kept on a
leash at least 6 feet
long
Fires: In fire rings
Alcohol: Prohibited
Vehicles: Two cars
per site
Other: Quiet hours
10 p.m.–8 a.m.;
gathering firewood
prohibited; limit 6
persons per site

the turnaround, site 50 invites tent campers to spread out. At the rear of these sites, the forest closes in and songbirds entertain, flittering about the woodland. There is a latrine across from site 49, but no water source is available in this section. Across from site 46 is the trail-head for the Dogwood Trail, which leads trekkers down to this state park's main attraction–Little Beaver Creek.

Back to the main campground road and near site 2 are a pit latrine and self-registration station with post-ed details regarding the park, campground, and any planned activities. A camp host (located on one of the electric sites near the registration station) is available during the summer season to answer questions. Across the road from the registration station are the sun shower and the amphitheater. The sites that line both sides of the road from the camp host's site to the dead end are spaced decently and are favored by campers with small RVs. Sites 32 and 33 are situated farther off the road's edge than neighboring sites. A playground is adjacent to the parking spaces for these two sites—the perfect sce-nario for tent-camping families with small children. Site 23 sits at the end of this second campground road, offer-ing its tenants an overlook of the valley cut by the Little Beaver Creek centuries ago.

The North Country Trail (NCT), a 4,175–mile hiking trail that stretches from North Dakota to New York, meanders through Beaver Creek State Park for 6.3 miles. The NCT includes various hiking challenges from creek crossings to roadside walks. Hiking at Bea-ver Creek should not be rushed; take time to pause and absorb the diverse sights and sounds. Remnants of his-toric river locks can be seen while maneuvering along the trail near the river. Before hikers reach the valley floor and Little Beaver Creek, the trail winds around the sides of forested ridges that warrant pauses to enjoy this special place.

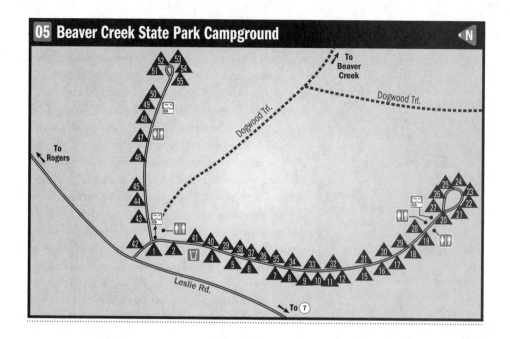

GETTING THERE

From East Liverpool, travel north on OH 11 for 5.45 miles to the OH 7 north exit. Follow OH 7 north for 2.98 miles to Leslie Road on the right. Go 0.81 mile to the campground entrance on the right.

GPS COORDINATES

N40°43.857'
W80°37.374'

6
BIG CREEK PARK

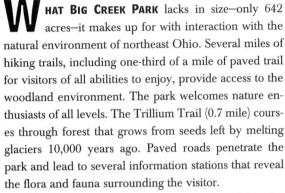

> *A small park with a big dose of natural exploration opportunities*

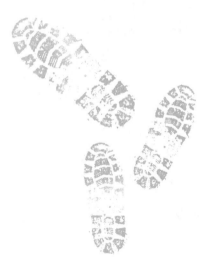

WHAT BIG CREEK PARK lacks in size—only 642 acres—it makes up for with interaction with the natural environment of northeast Ohio. Several miles of hiking trails, including one-third of a mile of paved trail for visitors of all abilities to enjoy, provide access to the woodland environment. The park welcomes nature enthusiasts of all levels. The Trillium Trail (0.7 mile) courses through forest that grows from seeds left by melting glaciers 10,000 years ago. Paved roads penetrate the park and lead to several information stations that reveal the flora and fauna surrounding the visitor.

Big Creek Park's four campsites are located in the park's northern region. As campsites go, this is about as good as it gets—especially because the park lies in the middle of a light residential area. While walking to these sites, you soon forget that neighborhoods and roads are less than a mile away. A gravel lane leads to a wide parking area, and a sign displays the campground's reservation schedule for the next few days. There is no guessing what site is what, and all regulations are clearly posted. The park's ponds, sitting, and wildlife viewing areas, as well as the trails leading to the park's intensely preserved natural surroundings, are all well maintained.

Sites A and B are found by walking 20 yards into the oak tree–dominated forest. Site A is first. It's not difficult to select a location for the tent, as two tent pads made of timber frames and filled with a bed of bark mulch mark the spot. The tent pads are approximately 12 feet by 16 feet and sit slightly aboveground to ensure a dry floor. The 8-foot-wide pathway that directs campers to these sites is well packed—using a small utility cart to wheel in your gear will not be a problem. At the entrance to site A sits a firewood rack with a raised bottom and covered roof. Firewood is not provided by the park system, but previous campers often leave leftover wood. The east edge of site A offers access to the Paw Paw hiking trail.

RATINGS

Beauty: ✿ ✿ ✿
Privacy: ✿ ✿ ✿
Spaciousness: ✿ ✿ ✿ ✿
Quiet: ✿ ✿ ✿ ✿
Security: ✿ ✿
Cleanliness: ✿ ✿ ✿

Site B sits 20 yards back from site A and has a similar layout to site A, with tent pads, fire ring with grate, and two picnic tables. Painted on a large oak tree at site B are blue blazes, guiding hikers working the section of the Buckeye Trail that slips through Big Creek Park. The Buckeye Trail is a 1,444-mile hiking circuit of trails and roads that wind around Ohio, touching each corner of the state.

Sites C and D can be accessed from the parking area using a separate path from A and B's pathway. Sites C and D don't have tent pads, but instead each site features a lean-to covered with cedar siding and roofing. The lean-tos each have full sides and a raised, wooden floor, allowing for a small dome tent inside. Rising in front of each lean-to is a stone chimney with a fireplace that faces the lean-tos' interior. Big Creek Park rules state that no cooking is to be done inside the fireplace; it is intended for heat and light only. A few feet of open space on either side of the chimney allow campers access into the lean-to.

Another park property that must be experienced is found by leaving Big Creek Park's entrance and traveling north for 0.36 mile to Pearl Road on the right. Follow Pearl Road for 0.84 mile to the parking area and trailheads of Whitlam Woods. Deep ravines decorated with multiple species of ferns and flora found only in northern habitats thrive here in this special park. Huge hemlocks, maples, and beech trees cover this 100-acre park, and a trail system gives entry to the mature forest that has escaped development over the last century. A photo-worthy trail descends to the cool bottom of a ravine and crosses a creek via a wooden footbridge. Pause on the bridge and study the creek for a glimpse of aquatic critters moving about the stones.

KEY INFORMATION

ADDRESS: 9160 Robinson Rd. Chardon, OH 44024

OPERATED BY: Geauga Park Dist.

INFORMATION: (440) 286-9516; www.geauga parkdistrict.org

RESERVATIONS: (440) 286-9516; www.geauga parkdistrict.org

OPEN: Year-round

SITES: 2 w/tent pads; 2 w/lean-tos

EACH SITE: Fire ring, grill, picnic table, firewood rack, lantern-holding post

ASSIGNMENT: Make reservations at least 3 days in advance

REGISTRATION: Permit must be kept on person; printable permit online; permit at Meyer Center on Big Creek Park grounds

FACILITIES: Latrines, water, fishing lake, pay phone at entrance to Meyer Center

PARKING: In parking area— a 40-yard walk to sites required.

FEE: Free for Geauga Cty. residents; $20 for nonresidents

ELEVATION: 1,119 feet

RESTRICTIONS: *Pets:* On leash only *Fires:* In fire ring *Alcohol:* Prohibited *Vehicles:* None *Other:* Camping by permit only; must be 18 to obtain a permit; cutting trees or gathering firewood prohibited

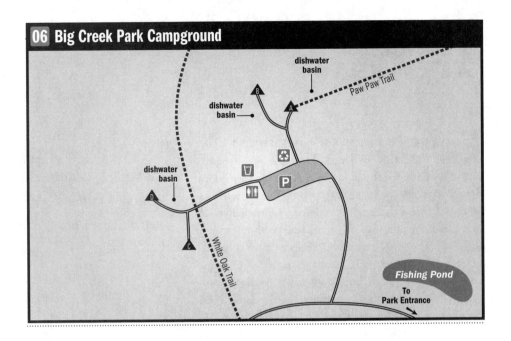

GETTING THERE

From I-90 take exit 200 south of Painesville; go south on OH 44 for 3.7 miles to Clark Road on the left. Travel east on Clark Road for 1.85 miles to Robinson Road on the right. Follow Robinson Road south for 0.87 mile to the park entrance on the right.

GPS COORDINATES

N41°37.289'
W81°12.051'

FERNWOOD STATE FOREST

EARLY SETTLERS ENTERING SOUTHEAST OHIO were met with steep hills and deep hollows covered with heavy forest. The area that makes up Fernwood State Forest today was one of the first to test the settlers. What was then a challenging wilderness is now a diverse and expansive landscape of woodlands, with meadows mixed in. The 2,107-acre state forest was once stripped of coal via surface mining, although hundreds of acres were left untouched. Those forest-covered ridges have matured into a woodland recreational area—some trees here are more than 100 years old. Not far from the Ohio River, the ridges and valleys under Fernwood are also evidence of the land-changing waters that flowed here thousands of years ago. Reforestation programs are ongoing, promising additional forest cover for generations to come. Fernwood State Forest's woodlands call to those who cherish the forest environment. The mining activities left behind dozens of ponds flanked with high wall cliffs (so watch your step when off-trail hiking), that now provide decent bass fishing. The forests are teeming with wildlife, managed with ethical hunting seasons. Fernwood is a popular destination for anglers, hunters, and ATV enthusiasts. ATV riders are restricted to designated areas, which keeps things calm and quiet for those who prefer to explore on foot.

Fernwood State Forest consists of four sections, each only a mile or so apart. Sitting atop a ridge in the forest's northern section is the Hidden Hollow Campground. Although the ridgeline location and the campground's name don't match, the "hidden" title is correct. A recently paved road welcomes campers to this concealed campground. Don't let the first glimpse of site 1 mislead you into thinking the sites are too small for a tent. The sites are not wide, but they are long, and each has a paved parking space. At the end of the parking space the campsite begins, tucked under shade trees and

> *Fernwood features healthy forestlands and expansive vistas.*

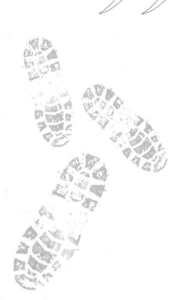

RATINGS

Beauty: ☆☆☆
Privacy: ☆☆☆
Spaciousness: ☆☆☆
Quiet: ☆☆☆☆
Security: ☆
Cleanliness: ☆☆☆

ADDRESS:	11 Township Rd. 181, Bloomingdale, OH 43910
OPERATED BY:	ODNR Division of Forestry
INFORMATION:	(740) 266-602; www.ohiodnr.com/DNN/forests/fernwood/tabid/5152/Default.aspx
RESERVATIONS:	First come, first served
OPEN:	Year-round
SITES:	22 primitive
EACH SITE:	Fire ring, picnic table
ASSIGNMENT:	First come, first served
REGISTRATION:	Campers must select a site; a forest officer will issue a permit
FACILITIES:	Pit latrine, waste water disposal basin, trash containers, hand water pump
PARKING:	At each site
FEE:	Free
ELEVATION:	1,180 feet
RESTRICTIONS:	*Pets:* Permitted *Fires:* In fire ring *Alcohol:* Prohibited *Vehicles:* 2 per site *Other:* Berries, nuts, and mushrooms may be gathered and removed, except from tree seed orchards or posted areas.

surrounded by wild shrubs and wildflowers. The picnic table, fire ring, and your tent are hidden from the road by your vehicle. Each site is also divided by small trees and vegetation, which add to the element of privacy.

The sites are situated along each side and around the cul de sac of the quarter-mile campground road. Sites 3 and 4 offer the most solitude when the campground gets busy, but that is hardly ever the case. During the deer hunting seasons in October and November, this campground serves as a base camp for sportsmen roaming the 3,000-acre state forest in search of Ohio's most sought-after game animal. At the end of the road, on the outside of the paved loop, are sites 9, 10, and 11. These sites are not as deep as the first eight, but they do provide ample tent space adjacent to the parking space. Inside the loop is the latrine—a clean, well-maintained facility. A bulletin board mounted to the front wall of the latrine holds a map of the forest. Hiking through the forest is primarily free hiking (there are no established trails). A designated trail is accessible between sites 17 and 18, where you'll also find a hand-operated water pump (nonpotable water). The hiking trail (no horses permitted), titled the Fernwood Land Lab Trail, showcases continuing forest, soil, and water management practices that involve area schoolchildren annually.

For an impressive overlook of the forest region, jump in the car and drive from the campground back to CR 26. From there, turn left (east) and travel 2.74 miles to the forest headquarters on a service road on the right. Follow this 1.5-mile dead end road that presents two scenic overlooks on the left. Near the end of this service road is a small picnic area that looks like a campground but isn't. The view at the overlooks is an awesome expanse of some of Ohio's steepest ridges and deepest ravines. After enjoying a picnic at one of the overlooks' many picnic tables, return to CR 26, turn right, and descend more than 300 feet in less than 0.75 mile. Drive slowly and enjoy the view as you traverse the steep ravine. At the end of CR 26, turn right and take to the next road on the left. This is Fernwood Road, and it leads to Wintersville, a medium-sized town with plenty of retail outlets to restock for the remainder of the camping trip.

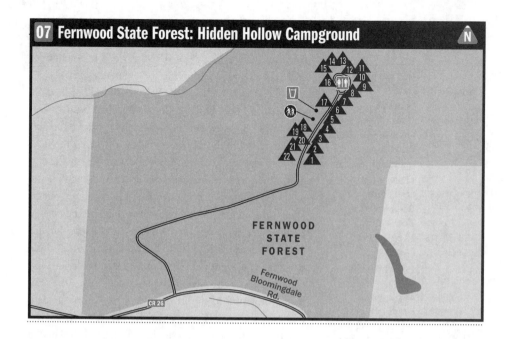

GETTING THERE

From Bloomingdale, follow CR 26 south 2.26 miles to where CR 26 and CR 25 converge. Turn left and stay on CR 26 for 0.72 mile to campground signage on the left and make a left turn onto the forest road. Travel 0.52 mile and turn left into the campground.

GPS COORDINATES

N40°19.863'
W80°45.966'

8
FINDLEY STATE PARK

This forestland retreat features a pleasing, calm lake in its center.

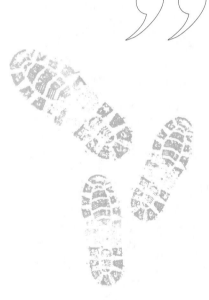

DISCOVERING THE FORESTED Findley State Park among the level agricultural lands of north central Ohio is a pleasant surprise. The park surrounds the 93-acre Findley Lake, an electric motors–only impoundment. Kayaking or canoeing the lake is a popular warm-weather pursuit and for worthy reasons: wildlife, birds, lake coves, and curvy shorelines, and a diversity of aquatic vegetation decorating it all. When snows blanket the park, hardy tent campers with cross-country skis enjoy this forest oasis and the manageable trails that wind and weave through the heart of the park.

Entering the park through its main entrance from OH 58 gives visitors the feeling they are passing through a geographical portal. Take a right and travel south on Park Road 3 to find the campground, not before passing through a challenging disc golf course 0.25 mile south of the park entrance. A camp office well stocked with supplies stands at the camp entrance and the first-come, first-served sites (1–27) can be found by turning right past the camp office onto Park Road 6.

This nonelectric section is the farthest from Findley Lake, the main attraction of Findley State Park. What this section does offer is a stay deeper in the forest. Site 3 sits back a dozen yards from the park road, while most of this campground's sites are at road's edge. Sites 14 and 15 are a pair of sites to accommodate a couple of camping families that want to interact but still appreciate a touch of privacy from neighboring sites. At the end of Park Road 6 is a cul-de-sac with site 26 being the choice of the few sites on the outside of the turnaround. Site 26 is roomy with space for a family-sized tent and plenty of room for folks to gab around the fire ring. Findley State Park's campground rule states that all tents must be placed within 30 feet of the parking pad—not a problem as the forest touches nearly all of the campground roads.

RATINGS

Beauty: ✩ ✩ ✩
Privacy: ✩ ✩
Spaciousness: ✩ ✩
Quiet: ✩ ✩
Security: ✩ ✩ ✩
Cleanliness: ✩ ✩ ✩

Halfway from Park Road 6 back to Park Road 3, on the right is Park Road 8 and sites 38–70. These sites are all nonelectric, which discourages RV owners from setting up in this quiet section. Site 57 touches the turnaround with a parking pad but sprawls out under a heavy tree canopy during the summer months and is sprinkled with orange and red leaves during the fall. This site will accommodate a few small tents as well as a dining canopy. Site 68 sits on the right as Park Road 8 nears the intersection with Park Road 6, a wider-than-average site with ample privacy on both sides.

Back to Park Road 3, turn right to find sites 72–120—all nonelectric. Although this section lies in the center of the campground, it still remains fairly quiet even during peak summer camping season. The 0.8-mile Spillway Trail passes between sites 84 and 85, leading trekkers to the dam and a wide view of the lake—a perfect spot to watch the sunset. Across the road at site 112, the 0.5-mile Lake Trail emerges from the forest. Lake Trail is an easy walk that presents a senses-pleasing blend of forest meets lake settings. As Park Road 3 returns to the main intersection, sites 124, 126, and 127 on the right are wooded sites with trees standing within several feet of each other—tight forest camping that creates a sense that you're off the beaten path. Just past these sites, turn right onto Park Road 11. Most of these sites are more open than the others, allowing direct sun to shine down during most of the day. Site 151 is a pleasing tent spot where the forest juts out towards the road.

Park Roads 12 and 13 hold the electric sites, so RVs are king in those two sections. But Park Road 10 is a 0.20-mile road that leads to the campground boat ramp—an easy access point to shove off your kayak. Sites 260–283 flank the road. Site 233 offers some privacy thanks to close trees and medium-sized shrubs. Site 279 is tucked back into the woods, and even though the boat ramp road sees some traffic, the site remains agreeable for tent camping.

The 200-acre Wellington Wildlife Area is a western neighbor of the state park. Directly across OH 58 is a wildlife area that includes two small ponds perfect for quiet fishing. The property hosts a healthy population of small game, such as cottontail rabbits and pheasants, for

KEY INFORMATION

ADDRESS:	25381 St. Rt. 58 Wellington, OH 44090-9010
OPERATED BY:	ODNR Division of State Parks
INFORMATION:	(440) 647-4490; www.dnr.state .oh.us/parks
RESERVATIONS:	(866) 644-6727; www.ohio.reserve world.com
OPEN:	Year-round; limited facilities in winter; heated showers and store closed Nov.–March
SITES:	181 nonelectric; 90 electric
EACH SITE:	Picnic table, fire ring
ASSIGNMENT:	Reservable sites; walk-in sites first come, first served
REGISTRATION:	Self-registration station at office, if office closed
FACILITIES:	Showers, flush toilets, laundry, camp store, sports courts, playground, swimming beach, boat rentals, disc golf course, nature center
PARKING:	At each site
FEE:	$23 nonelectric; $27 electric
ELEVATION:	914 feet
RESTRICTIONS:	*Pets:* On leash only *Fires:* In fire ring *Alcohol:* Prohibited *Vehicles:* 2 per site *Other:* Quiet hours 10 p.m.–8 a.m.; gathering firewood prohibited; limit 6 persons per site; checkout is 1 p.m.

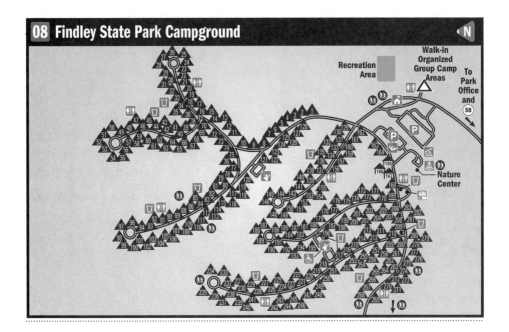

GETTING THERE

From Wellington, take OH 58 south 2.52 miles to the park entrance on the left. Follow Park Road #3 (and signage) on the right to the campground entrance.

hunters. Songbirds pause here during spring migrations, so bring your bird identification guide. Parking and a handicapped trail access are located on Griggs Road, which connects with OH 58 between the state park's main entrance and the park service area entrance 0.70 mile south of the main entrance.

Note: Campers must be 18 years old to rent a campsite.

GPS COORDINATES

N41°7.401'
W82°12.344'

HARRISON STATE FOREST

HARRISON STATE FOREST covers nearly 1,400 acres that were mined for coal in the late 1950s. Since the land was purchased by the state of Ohio in 1961, supporting a sustainable forest here was the objective, and that goal has been reached. Within this remote forestland are ponds of various sizes and trees that have grown to mature status. The reforestation projects continue today, following the Division of Forestry's long-term management plan. For outdoors enthusiasts, Harrison State Forest has grown into a rugged playground with miles of woodlands to explore.

There are two designated camping areas within the Harrison State Forest boundaries. One is an equestrian campground; the other is the Ronsheim Campground, a family camp. The Ronsheim Campground consists of seven sites spread around the side of a rounded ridge like a hand of playing cards. The paved lane that rolls through the campground seems out of place in such a remote campground, but because of the grounds' downward slope, the hard road is welcome. Sites 1–6 are on the left, on the low side of the hill. The sites are well spaced but a bit small, and site 4 has only space for a small tent. On the opposite side of the road from site 4 is a hand water pump; boil or filter the water before using.

Site 7 is also on the right side of the road, near the drinking water supply and latrine. Back across the road from site 7 is a trailhead identified with a brown sign displaying the word DAM. The trail descends 400 feet to a long but narrow remote lake surrounded by forest, except for the dam. Pack a rod and reel and a few plastic worms to catch the evening's dinner. Largemouth bass averaging two pounds are common in these surface mining reclamation ponds that are numerous throughout southeastern Ohio.

A bulletin board mounted on the latrine building posts information regarding camping at Harrison

Explore hundreds of acres of mature woodlands at Harrison State Forest.

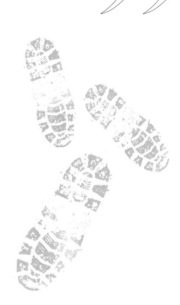

RATINGS

Beauty: ✿ ✿
Privacy: ✿ ✿ ✿
Spaciousness: ✿ ✿ ✿
Quiet: ✿ ✿ ✿ ✿
Security: ✿ ✿
Cleanliness: ✿ ✿

ADDRESS: Toot Road
Cadiz, OH 43907

OPERATED BY: ODNR's Division
of Forestry

INFORMATION: (740) 266-6021 (This
phone number
will reach admin-
istrative offices at
nearby Fernwood
State Forest);
www.ohiodnr.com/
DNN/forests/
harrison/tabid/
5155/Default.aspx

RESERVATIONS: First come,
first served

OPEN: Year-round

SITES: 7 primitive

EACH SITE: Fire ring,
picnic table

ASSIGNMENT: First come,
first served

REGISTRATION: Forest Officer will
visit occupied sites
and issue camping
permit

FACILITIES: Pit latrine, waste-
water disposal
basin, trash con-
tainers, hand water
pump

PARKING: At each site

FEE: Free

ELEVATION: 1,226 feet

RESTRICTIONS: *Pets:* Permitted
Fires: In fire ring
Alcohol: Prohibited
Vehicles: 2 per site
Other: Berries, nuts,
and mushrooms
may be gathered
and removed ex-
cept from tree seed
orchards or posted
areas.

State Forest and Ohio's State Forest system. This campground doesn't offer any organized activities or programs, but rather a quiet place to be enveloped by the forest's sights and sounds. If you see a large bird with a red crown and black-and-white striped face quickly flying from large tree to large tree, it may be Ohio's largest woodpecker, the Pileated Woodpecker. With the forest surrounding the campground, and without any residential buildings or homesteads nearby, the wildlife here is active year-round. It's your responsibility to blend in to take in the show.

From September through October, sports enthusiasts frequent the small campground. The entire Harrison State Forest attracts both hunters and anglers. There are a couple of sportsmen's clubs located on a neighboring road. Open to the public, a shooting and archery range is available on Township Road 182, the neighboring road. To get a good look at the forest's diversity, hit one of the forest's many marked hiking/bridle trails. From the campground, return to the entrance to the campground and go right on Toot Road. You'll reach a parking area at 100 yards, which is used by equestrians for parking their trucks and trailers. A trail leads to the west and meanders for 0.90 mile before arriving at and crossing TR 182. For even more miles of trekking adventure, turn north on TR 182 and go past the gun range to a continuation of the hiking/bridle trail, heading west for 1.07 miles to meet TR 186. Follow the trail across TR 186 and go 0.45 mile to the equestrian campground. The trail leads hikers and horses through pine and deciduous forests of various densities and skirts several ponds.

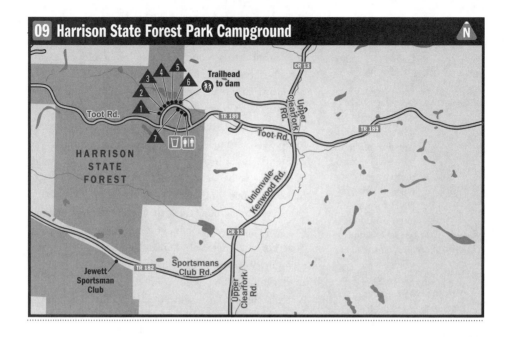

Trailhead
to dam

CR 13

Upper
Clearfork
Rd.

Toot Rd.

TR 189

Toot Rd.

TR 189

HARRISON
STATE
FOREST

Unionvale-
Kenwood Rd.

CR 13

Jewett
Sportsman
Club

TR 182

Sportsmans
Club Rd.

Upper
Clearfork
Rd.

GETTING THERE

From Cadiz, follow OH 9
north for 3.54 miles to CR 13
(Upper Clearfork Road) on
the right. Travel 2.26 miles to
TR 189 (Toot Road) on left.
Watch for a brown signpost
with a tree symbol at the corner of CR 13 and Toot Road.
Go 0.73 mile to the camp-
ground road on the right.

GPS COORDINATES

N40°19.803'
W80°59.375'

10
PORTAGE LAKES STATE PARK

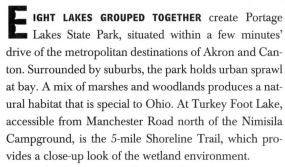

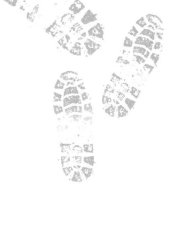

> *Portage Lakes State Park features more than 2,000 acres of water, with hundreds of species of wildlife thriving among it all.*

EIGHT LAKES GROUPED TOGETHER create Portage Lakes State Park, situated within a few minutes' drive of the metropolitan destinations of Akron and Canton. Surrounded by suburbs, the park holds urban sprawl at bay. A mix of marshes and woodlands produces a natural habitat that is special to Ohio. At Turkey Foot Lake, accessible from Manchester Road north of the Nimisila Campground, is the 5-mile Shoreline Trail, which provides a close-up look at the wetland environment.

The Nimisila Peninsula is a bird watcher's paradise, from eagles and ospreys, to warblers and purple martins. The purple martins perform quite an aerial show in the fall as they gather by the thousands to prepare for their migration south. Avid birders make a migration of their own to the Nimisila Peninsula to witness this impressive act of nature.

With so much natural splendor to observe, a quiet place to spend the night can be found at the small campground sitting on the peninsula in the middle of the Nimisila Reservoir, the southernmost lake of the Portage Lakes chain. The campground entrance is on the left before you reach the angler's parking area. From this parking area, several hundred yards of shoreline are accessible for anglers or bird-watchers. A small self-registration station stands at the campground gate, displaying posted information regarding the campground and the park. Because the park consists of several lakes and ponds—not all connected—having a map is a must to find your way around.

After passing by the campground information station, take a right to find the sites nearest to Nimisila Reservoir. The first thing on the right is a sun shower, a small wooden building rigged to hold a solar shower bag that you provide. It's a primitive way to wash, but it offers privacy to freshen up after a day of bird-watching or fishing. As you round the corner, the reservoir will

RATINGS

Beauty: ✿ ✿
Privacy: ✿ ✿
Spaciousness: ✿ ✿
Quiet: ✿ ✿ ✿
Security: ✿ ✿ ✿
Cleanliness: ✿ ✿

come into view through the few breaks in the forest. The campground is kept cool during the summer months by a mixed stand of pines and deciduous trees. Sites 14 and 16 sit near the lake's edge. These are deep and offer ample space for a tent close to the parking pad or closer to the lake. Just past site 16 is a teepee for rent.

The campground's elevation is not much higher than the reservoir's water level. Throughout the campground are several low spots that are somewhat marshy at times, although the campsites stay dry. Past the tepee near site 16 (there is another tepee on the campground road on the left after passing the sun shower) is site 24. Site 24 gives the best view of the lake and the surrounding boggy-like habitat. Don't be surprised if a Canada goose and a row of fuzzy goslings pass through the site during breakfast on a spring camping trip. Camping on the wild ones' turf adds to the unique camping experience of Portage Lakes State Park. Sites 41–52 pull away from the reservoir as the campground road turns back inland. After passing site 52, a boat launching ramp and small, sandy beach are on the right. As the road turns back to the campground entrance, sites 58–70 sit among a mature pine woodlot. These sites are well spaced and flank both sides of the road. Although the campground is not in a remote forest or miles away from any village, the Portage Lakes campground environment creates the sensation of an out-of-the-way place to stay.

KEY INFORMATION

ADDRESS:	5031 Manchester Road Akron, OH 44319
OPERATED BY:	ODNR Division of State Parks
INFORMATION:	(330) 644-2220; www.dnr.state .oh.us/parks
RESERVATIONS:	(866) 644-6727; www.ohio .reserveworld.com
OPEN:	Year-round; limited facilities in winter months, but water is available
SITES:	68 nonelectric; 6 electric
EACH SITE:	Fire ring, picnic table
ASSIGNMENT:	Reservable sites; walk-in sites first come, first served
REGISTRATION:	Self-registration at campground entrance station
FACILITIES:	Sun shower, latrines, sports courts, playground, camper's beach, potable water
PARKING:	At each site
FEE:	$22 nonelectric; $26 electric; $1 off Sunday–Thurs.; $2 off during winter
ELEVATION:	1,007 feet
RESTRICTIONS:	*Pets:* On leash only *Fires:* In fire ring *Alcohol:* Prohibited *Vehicles:* 2 vehicles per site, provided they are on paved pad; overflow parking available *Other:* Quiet hours 10 p.m.–8 a.m.; gathering firewood prohibited; limit 6 persons per site

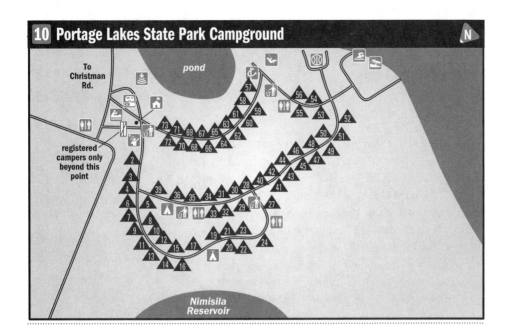

GETTING THERE

From I-77 Exit 111, north of Canton, go west on Portage Street 4.66 miles to Lutz Avenue on the right. Travel north on Lutz Avenue 2.07 miles to Mt. Pleasant Street. Turn right and then immediately left onto Christman Road and travel north 2.24 miles to the park entrance on the left.

GPS COORDINATES

N40°56.561'
W81°31.250'

11
PUNDERSON
STATE PARK

PUNDERSON LAKE is one of Ohio's few natural lakes— a "kettle lake" formed by a remaining chunk of a receding glacier—and is also the largest and deepest of these unique lakes in the state. Although the lake permits boat motors up to 20-hp, paddling is the preferred power source. The abundance of aquatic life skirting the lake's edges is best approached by gliding kayak. Throughout the park's surrounding woodlands, meadows, and marshes, wildlife—especially birds—are prevalent here. Stop at the bulletin board near the gazebo on the main park road to get an update on the park's bluebird population and see where the nesting boxes are. Punderson Lake State Park is truly a four-season recreation destination. The park's central trail, the Huron Trail, is trekked on by hikers and then slid across by cross country skiers when the snow falls. Since this park is smack in the middle of Ohio's snow belt, park visitors don't waste time waiting for summer.

Camping in the woods of Punderson Lake is a tradition of sorts. The campground overlays a former Native American village, so what is now a place of recreation was once a home for an ancient civilization. Tents are the favored means of lodging at Punderson—the dozens of "Tent Only" signs attached to the site identification posts confirms this.

The campground is basically split into two sections, north and south, and each offers a different flavor of camping style. The southern section rests at a lower elevation than its northern counterpart. From the campground office, turn right past the dump station. Pass the first sites and focus on sites 71 and 69 on the left at the road's end. These sites require a 10-yard jaunt up a slope to the sites in the edge of a young woodlot. Back in the car, turn left; sites 66 and 64 on the left are the same—perched on a hill and with level tent spots. Follow this road to another road with a dead

> *Punderson Lake is Ohio's largest natural lake.*

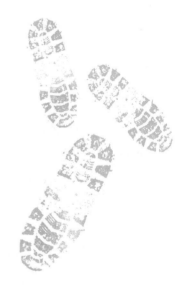

RATINGS

Beauty: ☆ ☆
Privacy: ☆ ☆
Spaciousness: ☆ ☆
Quiet: ☆ ☆
Security: ☆ ☆ ☆
Cleanliness: ☆ ☆

KEY INFORMATION

ADDRESS: 11755 Kinsman Rd. Newbury, OH 44065

OPERATED BY: ODNR Division of State Parks

INFORMATION: (440) 564-1195; www.dnr.state .oh.us/parks

RESERVATIONS: (866) 644-6727; www.ohio.reserve world.com

OPEN: Year-round; limited facilities winter

SITES: 12 nonelectric; 177 electric

EACH SITE: Picnic table, fire ring

ASSIGNMENT: Reservable sites; walk-in sites first come, first served

REGISTRATION: Self-registration if campground office closed

FACILITIES: Showers, flush toilets, laundry, sports courts, playground, swimming beach, boat rentals, marina, disc golf course, 18-hole golf course, archery range

PARKING: At each site

FEE: $22 nonelectric; $26 electric

ELEVATION: 1,154 feet

RESTRICTIONS: *Pets:* On leash only *Fires:* In fire ring *Alcohol:* Prohibited *Vehicles:* 1 per site unless a second can fit on parking pad; $2 per day fee for second vehicle *Other:* Quiet hours 10 p.m.–7 a.m.; gathering firewood prohibited; limit 6 persons per site; check out is 1 p.m.

end visible on the left. Stop at the dead end—a restroom is on the left, and off in the woods straight ahead are 8 primitive sites. These sites sit at the base of a hill and can be a touch muddy during wet weather. They also lack efficient space for a private night of tent camping.

From that dead end, turn around and drive through the number 40s sites. The road leads to the water treatment plant; turn right. Sites 26–15 are closest to Punderson Lake but elevated above the shoreline. Site 19 offers the best piece of land to place a tent and soak up the natural lake's aroma being carried by the gentlest breeze. Because of its nearly parallel angle to the road, site 19's parking pad serves as a privacy barrier when occupied by a vehicle. Place two chairs between the tent and the edge of the lake bank, and a seriously relaxing experience can be shared with a camping buddy.

To access the north section, return to the campground office and follow the camp road through sites 91–97. Site 96 parking is along the road, but the site is also on the peak of a small hill, surrounded by several small trees and low vegetation. Sites 100–156 are spotted along an ascending road to the highest point in the campground. Most of these sites are sunny and sloped. Back down the hill near site 99, the 156–201 area has a few tent-camping gems. Sites 187 and 188 are deep, wooded sites with several feet of vegetation between them and the next sites. The Erie Trail passes by these sites, offering a footpath to both Punderson Lake and Stump Lake—great destinations to observe various species of waterfowl in action.

Note: Persons under 18 years old must have written consent of parent or legal guardian to register for a campsite.

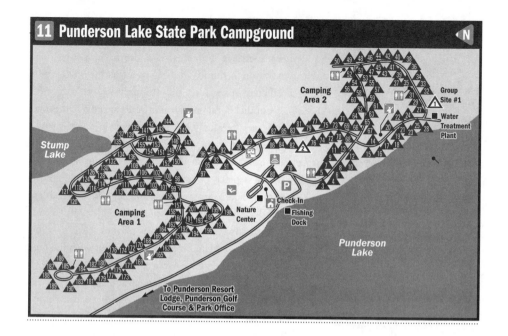

To Punderson Resort Lodge, Punderson Golf Course & Park Office

GETTING THERE

From Chardon, follow OH 44 south for 7.74 miles to OH 87. Turn right on OH 87 and go 1.51 miles to the park entrance on the left.

GPS COORDINATES

N41°27.367'
W81°12.334'

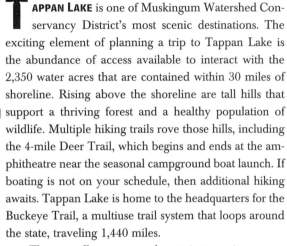

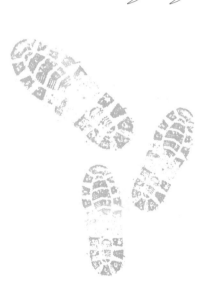

Tappan Lake is the ideal summer lake getaway destination.

TAPPAN **L**AKE is one of Muskingum Watershed Conservancy District's most scenic destinations. The exciting element of planning a trip to Tappan Lake is the abundance of access available to interact with the 2,350 water acres that are contained within 30 miles of shoreline. Rising above the shoreline are tall hills that support a thriving forest and a healthy population of wildlife. Multiple hiking trails rove those hills, including the 4-mile Deer Trail, which begins and ends at the amphitheatre near the seasonal campground boat launch. If boating is not on your schedule, then additional hiking awaits. Tappan Lake is home to the headquarters for the Buckeye Trail, a multiuse trail system that loops around the state, traveling 1,440 miles.

Three small campgrounds rest in two pine groves and on a ridge above the southern lagoon of Tappan Lake. Not far from the beach is the first of two primitive campgrounds, both offering a quiet reprieve from the marina and seasonal campground, which are busy with lake lovers through the summer. Mount a bike for an easy ride to the sandy beach or grab an ice-cream cone at the camp store near the seasonal campground entrance.

Primitive campground number one rests at a lower elevation to the other two campgrounds included in this profile. During wet spells, campground one remains damp with some slight pooling. The good news: That's the only negative of the campground system at Tappan Lake. Well-displayed signage directs campers to these campgrounds with ease. As you drive along the park road that follows the outer edge of the wide valley, look for primitive campground one on the right at the head of the valley. A small shelter house is on the left, as is a drinking water spigot. The 25 sites flank both sides of the paved road that ends with a tight loop that includes sites skirting its edge. The sites on the right going in have a small drainage ditch at the rear. Kids may find a few

RATINGS

Beauty: ✿ ✿
Privacy: ✿
Spaciousness: ✿ ✿
Quiet: ✿ ✿
Security: ✿ ✿
Cleanliness: ✿ ✿

crawdads clambering in and out of den holes in that little channel. Older white pine trees provide ample shade and whisper when the breeze blows. The two sites on the outer edge of the cul-de-sac, sites 814 and 815, offer quiet camping without close neighbors. Inside the cul-de-sac are pit latrines, a drinking water spigot, and a trash receptacle. Parking is on the grass—there's no stone or pavement—which may be muddy during rains.

To reach the second primitive campground, return to the main park road and turn right. Just around the bend you'll find this campground a bit higher and drier, although the sites are shorter. There is sufficient space between sites, but another drainage ditch and a rapidly ascending hillside keep the campsite set-up close to the road. Pines similar in size to those found in campground one tower over most of this campground as well, but the surrounding vegetation is much denser. Be sure to pack an ample supply of insect repellent. This second primitive camp is also laid out on both sides of a dead-end road. On the left side of the road, as you approach the site-free loop, are four sites (912–915) grouped together in a small clearing in the pine forest. This is the perfect set-up for a group of friends or family camping together. At the campground entrance there are a pit latrine and drinking water spigot.

Leave the second primitive camp and continue uphill on the main park road 0.45 mile to reach the next camp. On the left at the top of a ridge overlooking the lake, the Class B campground provides electric to all of its 23 sites. These sites are conducive to tent camping, but small pop-up and hard-sided RVs also use these sites. This campground sits in a partial clearing with sites lining each side of the road. The road traces the center of the ridge and ends at another turnaround. Just short of the cul de sac are a pit latrine, drinking-water fountain, and a dishwater disposal basin. The road takes a slight turn around a shallow, wooded ravine, which gives the next site, site 711, more privacy than any other site in the campground. Site 711 sits among the trees but not among other campers.

Take a morning walk from Class B campground's entrance to the trailhead on the other side of the park road. Turkey Ridge Trail is a 1.5-mile hiking trail that

KEY INFORMATION

ADDRESS:	84000 Mallarnee Rd. Deersville, OH 44693
OPERATED BY:	Muskingum Watershed Conservancy District
INFORMATION:	(740) 922-3649; www.mwcd.org/ places/parks/ tappan-lake-park
RESERVATIONS:	(740) 922-3649; tappan@mwcd.org
OPEN:	Year-round
SITES:	54 primitive; 23 day camping w/ electric
EACH SITE:	Fire ring, picnic table
ASSIGNMENT:	All sites reservable; first come, first served
REGISTRATION:	Campground entrance station
FACILITIES:	Camp store, latrines, drinking water, boat ramp, boat rentals, swimming beach
PARKING:	At each site
FEE:	$25; $20 Oct.–Apr.
ELEVATION:	915 feet
RESTRICTIONS:	*Pets:* Must be registered as campsite occupant; on leash, max 6 feet *Fires:* In fire ring *Alcohol:* Allowed, but not publicly *Vehicles:* 2 per site *Other:* Camping permits issued to persons age 18 and older; checkout time is 4 p.m.; quiet hours 11 p.m.–7 a.m.; gathering of fallen tree limbs for firewood allowed

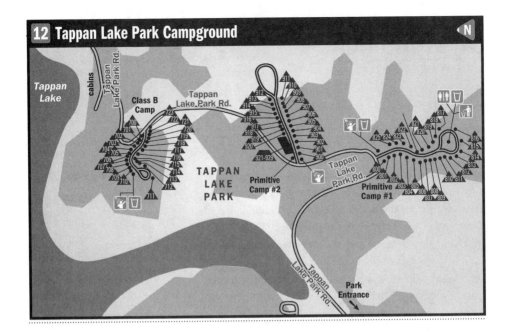

GETTING THERE

From Uhrichsville, follow OH 250 east 14.18 miles to CR 55 (Deersville Road) on the right. Travel 3.66 miles to Tappan Lake park entrance on the right. Follow signage to two primitive campgrounds.

leads to the Tappan Wetland Wildlife Area. This trail was developed by the National Campers and Hikers Association. At the observation station, listen and look for various waterfowl preparing to land through the fog rising off of the lake's warm water.

GPS COORDINATES

N40°19.139'
W81°10.708'

THE MAIN ATTRACTION at West Branch State Park is Michael J. Kirwan Lake. The lake's many coves and branches create perfect boating and angling opportunities. The 2,650-acre lake stretches over 7 miles, and its shoreline snakes around, leaving an abundance of forks and coves. Boating is the thing to do here, but if you have any energy left after your water fun, the park's 12 miles of hiking trails should polish off the day. A portion of the statewide Buckeye Trail passes through the park, including a 2-mile spur trail.

The lakeside camping here is first class, which is popular with campers who want to fish or dangle their feet in the water only a few steps from their campsite. West Branch's campground is spread out on a branched peninsula—four smaller peninsulas of various sizes joined together. Most of the campground is kept cool by mature deciduous trees. This popular campground receives a blend of visitors, and although it's busy, there are a few sites that yield quiet lakeside camping. The smallest and least busy section is also anchored to the smallest peninsula that rises 30 feet above the lake. Take the first right past the campground office to find this section. Sites 8–17 give wide views of the lake and provide plenty of shade. Sites 12 and 14 have steep, stone footpaths down to the water. At night, this section of the lake produces good catfishing action.

Backtrack to the main campground road and turn right to find sites 34–76. Sites 52 and 56 have broad views of the reservoir and access to the lake as well. This stretch of lakeside sites is popular with RVs, but there's ample space between sites and a focus on the lake view, which provides tranquility and makes this section appealing to tent campers too. At the tip of this long peninsula are sites 62 and 64, which are spacious and situated at the mouth of a lake cove. Site 62 slopes away from the road and down 20 yards to a bench—a perfect

> *Enjoy lake views and shoreline camping.*

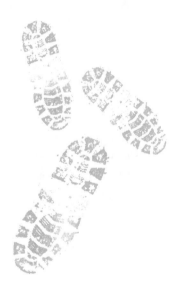

RATINGS

Beauty: ✩ ✩
Privacy: ✩ ✩
Spaciousness: ✩ ✩
Quiet: ✩
Security: ✩ ✩ ✩ ✩
Cleanliness: ✩ ✩

ADDRESS: 5708 Esworthy Rd.
Ravenna, OH
44266-9659

OPERATED BY: ODNR Division of
State Parks

INFORMATION: (330) 269-3239;
www.dnr.state
.oh.us/parks

RESERVATIONS: (866) 644-6727;
www.ohio.reserve
world.com

OPEN: Year-round;
limited facilities
in winter

SITES: 14 nonelectric; 155
electric; 5 ADA
sites

EACH SITE: Picnic table, fire
ring

ASSIGNMENT: Reservable sites;
walk-in sites first
come, first served

REGISTRATION: At camp office;
self-registration
station on front of
camp office

FACILITIES: Showers, flush toilets, laundry, sports
courts, playground,
swimming beach
near site 160, boat
rentals, pay phone

PARKING: At each site

FEE: $22 nonelectric;
$26 electric; $1 off
Sunday–Thursday;
$2 off during winter

ELEVATION: 1,013 feet

RESTRICTIONS: *Pets:* In designated
areas; on leash
only
Fires: In fire ring
Alcohol: Prohibited
Vehicles: 2 per site
Other: Quiet hours
10 p.m.–8 a.m.;
gathering firewood
prohibited; limit 6
persons per site

place to pitch a tent. A few steps more and you'll reach a gravel shoreline where you can launch a kayak or canoe. Just be sure to paddle early in the morning before the motorboaters rough up the lake's surface. Lakeside site 39 is ADA-accessible and situated across the lane from a heated shower house.

The central section of the divided peninsula is covered with sites 77–127. This segment includes several full-hookup sites for large RVs and is active with strolling campers on foot and on bikes. Avoid this area and head for the northwest peninsula branch, where you'll find sites 128–186. The nonelectric loop, sites 133–145, is mostly sunny and void of any views. Bypass that loop and go on to the two northern loops. The loop that includes sites 150–170 is separated from the bustling center of the campground. Site 160 is the site to behold—the best lakeside spot in the entire campground with a 180-degree view of the lake. The elevation is only a few feet different from the site to the lake. A buffer of vegetation and trees flanking both sides of the site make you feel as if you have the place to yourself. Just around the corner from site 160 is a small, sandy beach that doesn't get crowded.

A quiet loop next to the last hosts sites 171–186. Sites 180, 182, and 183 are also near the water's edge, at the mouth of a shallow cove with a view of the boat-launching ramp on the opposite side. These sites are less roomy but adequate for peaceful tent camping. After exiting that loop and heading toward the campground office, you'll encounter a row of sites worthy of consideration along a separate lane. Sites 187–198 include a few sites on the edge of a lake cove. Of those, site 193 provides the most solitude and best location for a shore lunch. Good numbers of crappie and walleye populate Michael J. Kirwan Lake and are available for filling your menu.

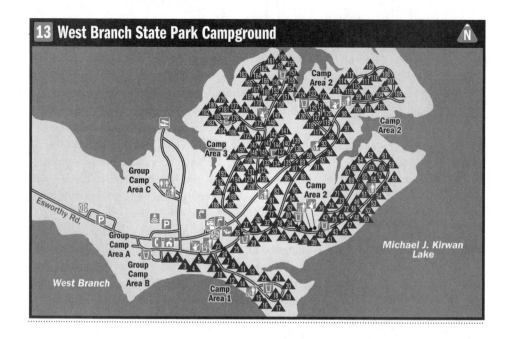

GETTING THERE

From I-76 Exit 38, south of Ravenna, travel north on OH 44 for 4.43 miles to where OH 44 blends into OH 5. Follow OH 5 for 3.03 miles east to Rock Spring Road on the right. Travel 0.3 mile to the park entrance on the left, and then on to the campground entrance.

GPS COORDINATES

N41°8.652'
W81°7.787'

14
WOODBURY
WILDLIFE AREA

Woodbury Wildlife Area offers an abundance of wildlife and solitude.

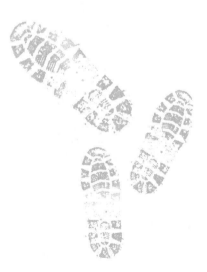

DESIGNATED WILDLIFE AREAS in Ohio hold some of the most remote, diverse wilderness that was once used for logging or mining. Successful reclamation efforts have resulted in thousands of acres for the public to explore and enjoy. No matter what your favored outdoor pursuit, an Ohio wildlife area can provide it. Woodbury Wildlife Area (WWA) is one such area, and it offers primitive camping possibilities as well. WWA comprises nearly 15,000 acres in its boundaries and is easily accessible via the multiple state routes that intersect the wild lands. More than 100 ponds lie in the maze of deep and shallow ravines—water impoundments created by the strip mining of coal during the early 1960s and 1970s. Visitors can explore the WWA by car or on foot. If you roam the ridges and hollows on foot, do so with care, as highwalls left by the mining still exist. Most footpaths that leave from the many roadside parking spots normally lead to a pond. Fishing these reclamation ponds rewards the remote angler with trophy-size gamefish, primarily largemouth bass. You must have four items in your daypack when hiking this backcountry: food, water, a map, and an orienteering device (compass or GPS). When you start maneuvering through the forest that covers the majority of the WWA, it's easy to mistake one trail for another on the return to the car or campsite.

Driving to the WWA primitive campground on TR 56, you will pass brushy fields on both sides of the road. These fields are managed by the Division of Wildlife for wildlife habitat. Mowed trails cut through these fields are primarily to provide hunters access and shooting lanes, but they also provide great wildlife-viewing pathways during the closed hunting seasons. A small folding camp stool is a perfect perch for sitting low along one of these mowed trails with camera in hand. In spring wild turkey is in season for hunters, but during the summer months, the big

RATINGS

Beauty: ✩ ✩
Privacy: ✩ ✩
Spaciousness: ✩ ✩
Quiet: ✩ ✩ ✩
Security: ✩
Cleanliness: ✩

birds and their white and red heads offer beautiful color contrast against the green foliage—time for another photo. The next target on the wildlife photo shoot list is the white-tailed deer. This animal is probably photographed more than any other wildlife species, but during the hunting off-season, catching a deer standing on the side of a ridge or sipping water from a pond in the early morning sunlight, antlers covered in velvet, is a worthy pose.

Approximately a quarter mile before arriving at the primitive campground, you will pass an old building with several doors on the left. This old shop is not in use, but the parking lot is used as an overflow lot when the primitive campground is full—mostly during fall hunting season. Both camping areas are supplied with portable latrines, but there's no drinking water at either one at any time of the year. Soon after passing the old shop, a small lake appears on the left. Watch for a few mallards to take flight if you pull into the small parking area that has a gravel ramp for launching small boats. The forested ridge on the opposite side of the lake is a candidate for that early-morning deer photo opportunity. This lake is wider and much more accessible than most of the waters in the WWA. Continuing on TR 56, you will see the campground lying at the base of the ridge to the right. The nine sites are not marked by signposts or any other marking. The sites are basically nine parking spaces with a 20-foot-wide grassy area in between each one. All sites are equal in dimensions and quality. They're as primitive as they come, except for the gravel access road. During closed hunting seasons, you may see only a couple of other campers while spending time at this campground and exploring the wildness of the place. If solitude is what you're after, the WWA can provide it. Several township, county, and state roads make access throughout the WWA simple. State Route 541 runs east and west through the heart of the WWA.

KEY INFORMATION

ADDRESS: 23371 SR 60 South Warsaw, OH 43844

OPERATED BY: ODNR Division of Wildlife

INFORMATION: (740) 824-3211; www.dnr.state.oh.us

RESERVATIONS: First come, first served

OPEN: Year-round

SITES: 9; overflow camping permitted nearby at old shop

EACH SITE: No amenities

ASSIGNMENT: First come, first served

REGISTRATION: None required

FACILITIES: Portable latrines

PARKING: At each site

FEE: Free

ELEVATION: 899 feet

RESTRICTIONS: *Pets:* Allowed on leash

Fires: Permitted

Alcohol: Permitted

Vehicles: No parking restrictions

Other: Vehicles must remain on roadways; camping in designated area only; no camping more than 6 consecutive days in a 30-day period; no generator use 10 p.m.–6 a.m.; must not leave site unattended more than 24 hours; minor supplies available in Warsaw; major supplies available in Coshocton

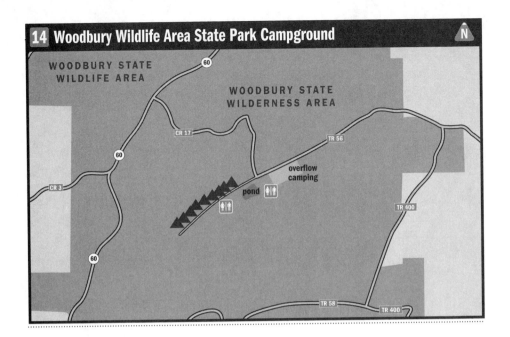

GETTING THERE

From Warsaw, take OH 60 south 2.39 miles to CR 17 on the left. Follow CR 17 1.03 miles to TR 56 on the right. Campground is located at the dead end in 1.06 miles.

GPS COORDINATES

N40°16.971'
W82°1.710'

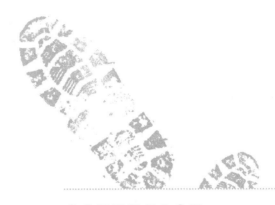

SOUTHEAST

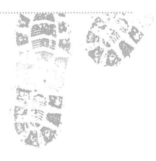

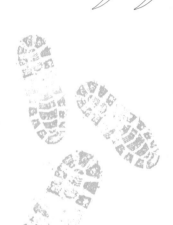

THE GIANT RUSTY BUCKET of the huge dragline named the Big Muskie is the only remaining remnant of the massive machine that extracted coal from southeastern Ohio's surface beginning in 1969. Today, 30,000 acres of those reclaimed mining lands, named the American Electric Power ReCreation Land (AEPRL), provide outdoors enthusiasts with a plethora of adventure. The land holds more than 350 ponds and lakes, a mix of deciduous and evergreen forests, rolling plains, and six campgrounds offering a variety of tent-camping scenarios. Although two interstate highways are within a short drive east and north, the AEPRL is one of Ohio's most remote camping destinations.

The six campgrounds are spread across the AEPRL and have individual characteristics, such as lakefront acreage (bring the kayak or canoe) or secluded, wooded creekside sites. Driving south on OH 83 from Cumberland, turn east on TR 13, and the first campground you'll encounter is Campground K. The drive alone quickly shakes the hustle-bustle feeling of a busy lifestyle as the

AEPRL offers remote camping and thousands of water acres for kayaking.

RATINGS

CAMPGROUND K (BICENTENNIAL)	CAMPGROUND D (SAWMILL ROAD)	CAMPGROUND G (MAPLE GROVE)
Beauty: ☆ ☆ ☆	Beauty: ☆ ☆	Beauty: ☆ ☆
Privacy: ☆ ☆ ☆	Privacy: ☆ ☆	Privacy: ☆ ☆
Spaciousness: ☆ ☆ ☆ ☆	Spaciousness: ☆ ☆	Spaciousness: ☆ ☆
Quiet: ☆ ☆ ☆	Quiet: ☆ ☆	Quiet: ☆ ☆
Security: ☆ ☆	Security: ☆ ☆	Security: ☆ ☆
Cleanliness: ☆ ☆ ☆	Cleanliness: ☆ ☆ ☆	Cleanliness: ☆ ☆ ☆
CAMPGROUND H (WOODGROVE)	**CAMPGROUND A (HOOK LAKE)**	**CAMPGROUND C (SAND HOLLOW)**
Beauty: ☆ ☆	Beauty: ☆ ☆ ☆	Beauty: ☆ ☆ ☆
Privacy: ☆ ☆	Privacy: ☆ ☆	Privacy: ☆ ☆ ☆
Spaciousness: ☆ ☆	Spaciousness: ☆ ☆ ☆	Spaciousness: ☆ ☆ ☆
Quiet: ☆ ☆	Quiet: ☆ ☆ ☆	Quiet: ☆ ☆ ☆
Security: ☆ ☆	Security: ☆ ☆	Security: ☆ ☆
Cleanliness: ☆ ☆ ☆	Cleanliness: ☆ ☆ ☆ ☆ ☆	Cleanliness: ☆ ☆

KEY INFORMATION

ADDRESS: P.O. Box 328,
McConnelsville, OH 43756

OPERATED BY: American Electric Power and Ohio DNR

INFORMATION: (740) 962-1205 or (800) WILDLIFE; www.aep.com/environmental/recreation

RESERVATIONS: First come, first served; must have a free AEP ReCreation Land permit (see details at the end of this profile)

OPEN: Primarily open year-round, but some close for winter

SITES: 176; overflow camping is permitted alongside designated sites within campgrounds

EACH SITE: Picnic table, fire ring (stone), trash can

ASSIGNMENT: First come, first served

REGISTRATION: At all campground entrance stations

FACILITIES: Pit latrines, potable water stations, information stations

PARKING: At each site

FEE: Free, but must have AEP ReCreation Land permit in possession

ELEVATION: Campground K: 866 feet; Campground H: 763 feet; Campground D: 831 feet; Campground A: 889 feet; Campground G: 954 feet; Campground C: 871 feet

RESTRICTIONS: *Pets:* On leash
Fires: In fire ring
Alcohol: Prohibited
Vehicles: No limits
Other: No cutting of live trees for firewood, but dead wood on the ground may be used; wading, bathing, and swimming are prohibited; no camp store; supplies available in Cumberland and McConnelsville

casually rugged land appears. The huge, colorful campground sign (all of the AEPRL campgrounds have these signs) is on the left. Turn left and follow the gravel road to and through the campground. The self-registration station is on the right. Once in the campground, a few unnumbered sites (no sites are numbered in the AEPRL campgrounds) in the open are on the right and offer plenty of space for multiple tents. The only pit latrine is also on the right.

After reaching the northernmost point of Campground K, the road turns west, then south, and follows the shoreline of a beautiful long and narrow lake. A potable water pump is available here. The first three campsites along the lake provide no shade, but access to the lake is only a couple of steps away. These lake sites offer plenty of elbow room between them—about 50 feet. Fishing in the AEPRL is popular year-round, especially for bass anglers. Be sure to include a heavy test line in your reel before casting to these largemouths that regularly weigh more than 4 pounds. Before the bottom lake road reconnects to the entry road, two sites on the right sit back in a wooded lot and offer easy lake access.

Back at the Campground K sign on TR 13, turn right and return to OH 83. To visit Campground H, turn south on OH 83 and go 1.4 miles to CR 27. Turn left and travel 2.6 miles to Campground H on the right. You will cross a creek on CR 27 before turning into the campground. This creek flows through the campground, offering kids the opportunity to flip over a few rocks in search of aqua critters. Soon after entering the campground, a group of eight sites are bordered by the entry and exit gravel lanes. These sites are heavily shaded and

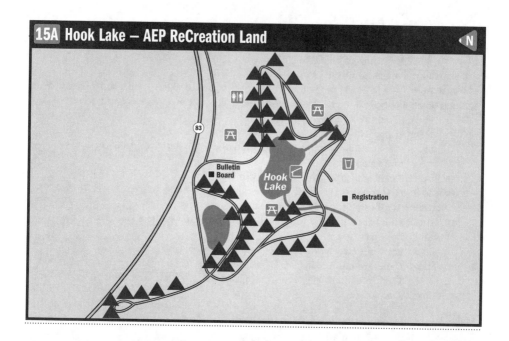

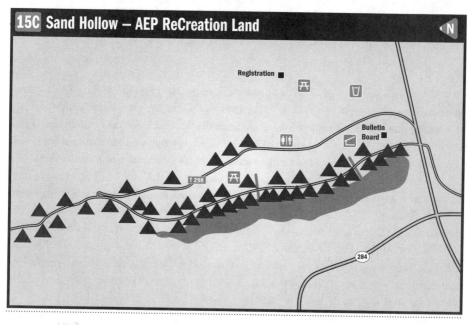

level, with a pit latrine available a few steps across the lane. As the lane leads into a wooded grove, the sites on the right are closer together, but all are creekside. The wooded grove gives a sense of tranquility, even with sites only 20 feet apart. The 16 sites along the creek are level, and space is available for a tent, though not a large one. Across the lane from the creekside

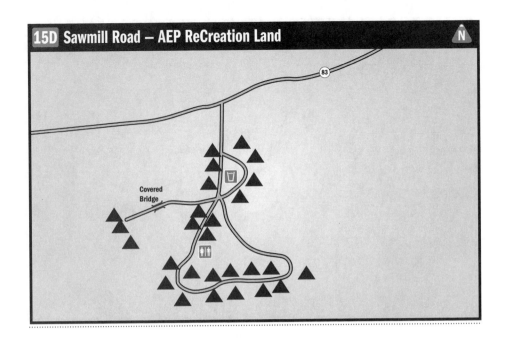

Covered
Bridge

sites are five level sites. A tent-only site (the only site on the right as the exit lane nears CR 27) is fairly open with shade on two sides. A camp host is on site in spring, summer, and fall.

A short walk southeast from the campground's entrance on CR 27 leads to access to the Buckeye Trail, a hiking trail that meanders around Ohio. At first, the trail was envisioned as a trail leading from the Ohio River to Lake Erie, but it evolved into a 1,444-mile trail offering hikers a path through Ohio's geographic diversity. The Buckeye Trail utilizes county roads, abandoned railroads, farmlands, and remote forests such as the section of trail that snakes through the AEPRL. The AEPRL section of the Buckeye Trail provides access to road-free areas of the AEPRL, but be careful, as hundreds of highwalls (cliffs) remain from the mining operations. Some of these have a drop of 50 feet or more, so it's important to stay on designated trails. Follow the blue blazes on trees and signposts.

To find Campground D, follow CR 27 back to OH 83. Take a short break once you reach the scenic overlook on OH 83, as there you will find more information regarding the AEPRL reclamation efforts and successes at a small park next to the AEPRL maintenance headquarters. You may also have some cellular phone service at this spot, as the elevation is 1,047 feet, one of the highest points in the area. After reading the history of the scene across the wide valley at the information station, travel south on OH 83 for 0.66 mile to the Campground D sign and access lane. The lane dead-ends at the campground. A few sites on the right approaching the main campground area offer privacy and young shade trees. A bit farther, on the left, are a volleyball court and swings with two sites nearby. Taking the right fork in the lane leads to wide, level sites on the left and a covered bridge on the right. The covered bridge is for foot traffic only and leads to a few secluded sites less than 50 yards from the bridge.

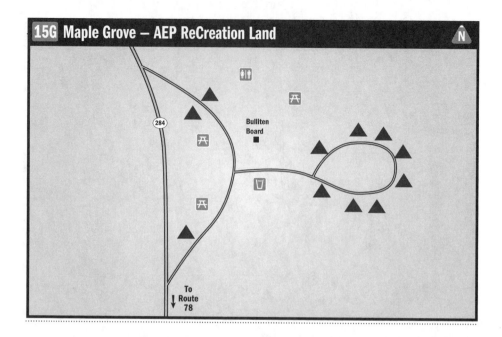

15G Maple Grove – AEP ReCreation Land

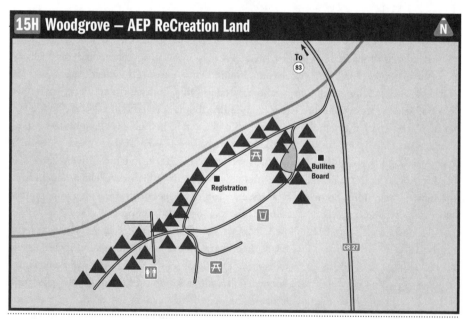

15H Woodgrove – AEP ReCreation Land

The second section of Campground D is uphill through a pine forest with sites on both sides of the lane. Each site is tent friendly, especially those on the right. At the top of the hill is a supply of sawmill slabs cut into sections for firewood (free for the taking). The lane turns back toward the camp entrance at the firewood center, passing a shelter house and camp host site on the way out. A short walk west of the covered bridge, two ponds await anglers and wildlife watchers.

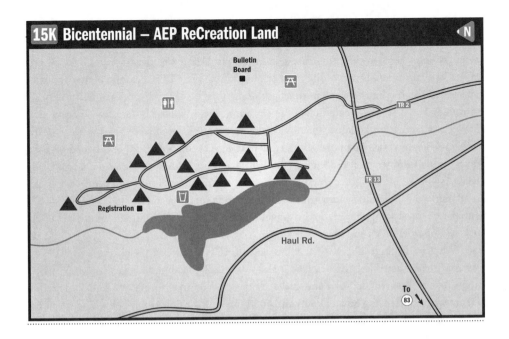

Bulletin
Board

TR 2

TR 13

Registration

Haul Rd.

To
83

Back at OH 83, turn left and go 1.7 miles to Campground A. Campground A is one of the largest of the six AEPRL campgrounds and possibly the nicest. Hook Lake is the main attraction here and is restricted for youth fishing only (anglers ages 16 and under). The lake is stocked occasionally with bass by conservation clubs and the ODNR's Division of Wildlife. The Hook Lake location also has a large, modern shelter house that is the site of several events during the year. During those times and holidays, Campground A gets busy. But at other times, the AEPRL campgrounds are fairly uncrowded. The southern section of Campground A is attractive to group campers such as Boy Scout troops. Those sites are open with very little shade but are spaced well apart, with more than 50 feet between them. In Campground A's northern section, sites are much smaller but situated in a forest surrounding three sides of Hook Lake. A few sites offer a narrow view of the lake. The lane leading through the northern section begins and ends near the campground entrance. The most tent-friendly sites lie on the left side of that looping lane. Bluebird boxes have been placed around the campgrounds, just as other wildlife attractions exist throughout the AEPRL, such as wildflower plantings and mowed pathways.

Moving along to Campground G, follow OH 83 south from Campground A for 2.15 miles to the intersection with OH 284. Turn right on OH 284 and go 0.14 mile to the Campground G entrance. Campground G, situated on top of a wooded knoll, is the smallest of the six AEPRL campgrounds. With only nine sites, it is mostly quiet except for the road noise that is nearby and within sight. Miner's Memorial Park, a must-see while in the AEPRL region, is only 0.7 mile south of Campground G. Follow OH 284 south until it blends with OH 78, and the park is on the right. Check out the Big Muskie's bucket on display there. The dragline's bucket weighs 460,000 pounds empty, and its volume equals a 12-car garage. An extensive informational display completes a visit to the park.

From Campground G, go north on OH 284 for 2 miles to Campground C's sign. Turn right onto the gravel road and follow it 0.4 mile to the entrance of Campground C. The campground stretches along the east side of a typical long and narrow reclaimed mining lake. Campground C is one of the most popular of the six AEPRL campgrounds, but with 50 sites spread out like gems on a stretched, straight necklace for 2.3 miles, it never appears crowded. The first mile, beginning at the entrance, skirts the lake's edge. The first five sites have direct access to the lake, which makes them tough to get unless you arrive before the weekend begins. Traveling north on the gravel road, sites on both sides of the road get a bit dusty in the summer months. Sites on the left have trails leading down a steep bank to the lake. As you follow the gravel road farther north, the number of sites tapers off. A T in the road marks the end of the campground. Turn around and proceed back to Campground C's entrance. Once there, turn left on the gravel road and follow it 1.4 miles to return to OH 83 near Campground A's entrance.

Whether fishing, hiking, or wildlife-viewing is your desire, it's all there at AEPRL. As you travel about the AEPRL, take it slow, as wildlife is abundant and regularly makes appearances—both on the road and at the campsites. You may even see a buffalo or zebra. Ok, maybe not crossing next to your tent, but those animals do exist at The Wilds, a wildlife conservation facility dedicated to rare and endangered species located within a few minutes' drive north of the campgrounds. The 10,000-acre center is the site of scientific studies and preservation practices of numerous species. Guided tours are available May–October. To visit The Wilds: From Campground C, take OH 284 8 miles north to International Road, turn right, and go one mile to the parking lot.

Note: You must have a free AEP ReCreation Land permit to camp in this area. Permits are available by calling (740) 962-1205 or (614) 716-1000, or by visiting **www.aep.com/ environmental/recreation/recland/permit.aspx.** They're also available at regional sporting goods or bait stores surrounding the ReCreation Land. A detailed map comes with the permit.

GETTING THERE

From I-70 Exit 169, take OH 83 south 11.4 miles to Cumberland. Continue south on OH 83 6.6 miles to TR 13. Turn left and follow TR 13 1.3 miles to Campground K entrance road on the left.

GPS COORDINATES

CAMPGROUND K:	CAMPGROUND A:
N39°46.198'	N39°43.672'
W81°38.414'	W81°42.478'
CAMPGROUND H:	CAMPGROUND G:
N39°43.282'	N39°42.367'
W81°40.202'	W81°43.527'
CAMPGROUND D:	CAMPGROUND C:
N39°44.673'	N39°44.037'
W81°41.477'	W81°43.864'

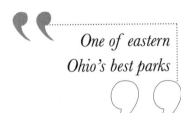

*One of eastern
Ohio's best parks*

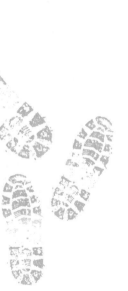

THE HILLS OF BELMONT COUNTY were frequented by settlers during the early 1800s, whose presence often caused conflicts with the Native Americans. The Native Americans treasured their land and rightly so. Still today, the beauty of the region and the bounty of natural resources is abundant here, and it is evident why so many people wanted to claim this region as their own. After the settlers became regular inhabitants of the then–heavily forested area, logging became a lucrative business. Barkcamp State Park gets its name from the de-barking facility that operated here a century ago, prepar-ing logs for transport. Inside the campground is a display of those pioneer days, complete with a variety of build-ings and antique implements. A paved trail titled Pio-neer Hiking Trail guides visitors through the collection of historical pieces. This trail is wheelchair-accessible, as are the campground's showers and restrooms. Paus-ing next to the hand-hewn log cabin and horse-drawn wagon parked next to it, one can imagine the work that went on here decades ago. Interpretive signs around the pioneer displays reveal some interesting facts. The park has received several awards for its cleanliness and the staff's dedication to delivering exceptional service, mak-ing it worthy of multiple visits.

A 117-acre lake is the park's focal point. Belmont Lake has an electric motor-only regulation; of course, paddling is allowed, and recommended. To find the boat ramp on the small lake, leave the campground and turn right, following posted signs. The view of the lake on the right is worthy of a quick stop to capture a photo before unloading the kayak or canoe—both of which can be rented here.

The first groups of campsites you come to while driving through the campground are often used by RV-ers, and the equestrian sites are in a loop on the right. Tents are welcome on these sites, but the best tent sites

RATINGS

Beauty: ☆ ☆ ☆
Privacy: ☆ ☆
Spaciousness: ☆ ☆
Quiet: ☆ ☆
Security: ☆ ☆ ☆ ☆
Cleanliness: ☆ ☆ ☆ ☆

are yet to come. Continue on the main road to camping area C. At the end of the road in camping area C are sites 122–134, the tent area. These sites are evenly spaced around the base of a round knoll approximately 50 yards in diameter. A young forest with a carpet of underbrush is laid out in a loop like a circle of wagons gathered in defense mode around these sites. Sites 125 and 131 give the most privacy to tent campers, as they are the farthest from the parking area. A restroom and drinking water spigot are located two sites away from the tent area on the main campground road. A connecting trail leaves the campground at the tent area and leads to a bridle/snowmobile trail that parallels the lake's shoreline and length of the entire campground. Though Barkcamp's hiking trails are short and total less than 4 miles, equestrian trails meander for more than 30 miles. Take one of the bridle trails for a trek on foot, but watch your step for spent horse fuel.

A special forest not far from the park is a must-see. Dysart Woods is a 50-acre tract of old-growth oak forest and the largest known remnant of the original forest of southeastern Ohio. Some of the trees here are more than 300 years old and stand 140 feet tall. The property is managed and studied by Ohio University. Two-foot trails wind through the old forest for visitors to explore, but not to touch or disturb the extraordinary natural environment. To find Dysart Woods, return to OH TR 92 and turn left. Drive 1.38 miles to OH 149 and turn right. Go 0.73 mile to OH 147 and turn left (south). Follow OH 147 for 4.79 miles to a wood Dysart sign on the right. A rustic restroom is located next to a white farmhouse on the left and parking is at the trailheads.

If you need to make a run for major supplies, your best bet is St. Clairsville.

KEY INFORMATION

ADDRESS: 65330 Barkcamp Park Rd., Belmont, OH 43718-9733

OPERATED BY: ODNR Division of Parks

INFORMATION: (740) 484-4064; www.dnr.state.oh.us/parks

RESERVATIONS: (866) 644-6727; www.ohio.reserveworld.com

OPEN: Year-round; limited water and facilities in winter

SITES: 150 electric; 27 equestrian sites

EACH SITE: Picnic table, fire ring

ASSIGNMENT: Reservable sites; walk-in sites first come, first served

REGISTRATION: At camp office; self-registration station on front of camp office

FACILITIES: Showers, flush toilets, laundry, payphone, playground, sports courts, boat ramp, boat rental, nature center, putt-putt golf, archery range

PARKING: At each site, but tent-only sites have a parking area

FEE: $20

ELEVATION: 1,225 feet

RESTRICTIONS: *Pets:* On sites 1–99 and on leash only *Fires:* In fire ring *Alcohol:* Prohibited *Vehicles:* 2 per site *Other:* Quiet hours 10 p.m.–7 a.m.; gathering firewood prohibited; 14-day stay limit; limit 6 persons per site

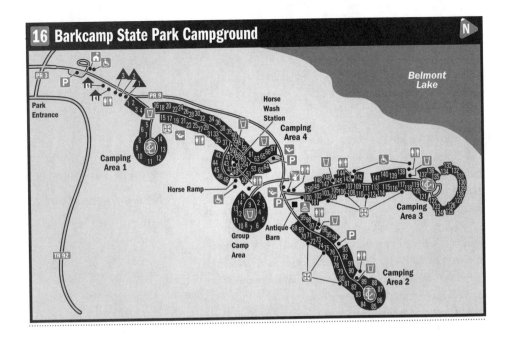

GETTING THERE

From I-70 Exit 208, north of Belmont, go south 0.8 mile on OH 149 to TR 92 on the left. Drive 0.93 mile to the park entrance on left. After entering the park, take an immediate right and follow to the campground entrance.

GPS COORDINATES

N40°2.780'
W81°1.767'

17
BLUE ROCK
STATE PARK

THE DRIVE TO THE PARK from the state route soon imparts a sense of tranquil serenity. A couple miles before arriving at the park's entrance, Blue Rock State Forest welcomes you. Towering pines close to the road blend with deciduous forest plots, creating a patchwork of colorful woodlands. At the park, the forests open up to reveal Cutler Lake, only 15 acres in size but overflowing with beauty with the towering forest as a backdrop. The lake was created in 1938 and remains the feature of this 322-acre gem of a state park.

There are two primary campgrounds at Blue Rock State Park, both located on the western side of the lake. The north campground (with 47 sites) lies below the lake's dam, with the spillway creek flowing through the heart of the campground, which makes a cool and soothing sound attraction for campers. The south campground (with 49 sites) is situated on a ridge and features some sites overlooking the lake. From the camp store, which is easily found on Cutler Lake Road on the north side of the lake, go back north on Cutler Lake Road 0.2 mile to the entrance of the north campground.

The north campground drive has a one-way pattern. Sites 52–56 are circled in a loop on the right. Behind and above these sites is Cutler Lake Road, and some road noise may steer tent campers to another site, but the traffic on the road is normally light. At the entrance to this loop you will find a bathroom and payphone. Following the one-way, paved lane, sites 59–64 are along the creek near a bridge that crosses the creek to a visitor's parking lot. These six sites offer the most privacy for the tent camper. The lane then follows a straight stretch of creek with sites between the lane and the creek and on the opposite side of the lane. Creek sites 66, 68, 70, 72, 74, 76, and 80 are walk-in sites. With Ohio State Parks, a walk-in site is one that is not reservable and is available for a camper that walks in to the registration

> *A small state park blessed with a huge dose of nature and tranquility.*

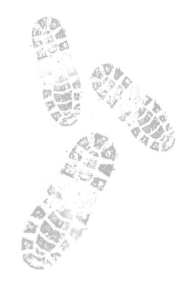

RATINGS

Beauty: ☆ ☆ ☆
Privacy: ☆ ☆
Spaciousness: ☆ ☆
Quiet: ☆ ☆ ☆
Security: ☆ ☆
Cleanliness: ☆ ☆ ☆

ADDRESS: 7924 Cutler Lake Rd., Blue Rock, OH 43720-9728

OPERATED BY: ODNR Division of State Parks

INFORMATION: (740) 453-4377 (This number will reach Dillon State Park, which handles Blue Rock's calls); www.dnr.state .oh.us/parks

RESERVATIONS: (866) 644-6727; www.ohio.reserve world.com

OPEN: Year-round; limited facilities in winter

SITES: 96 nonelectric

EACH SITE: Picnic table, fire ring

ASSIGNMENT: Reservable sites; walk-in sites first come, first served

REGISTRATION: At camp store; check in 3 p.m., check out 1 p.m.

FACILITIES: Camp store, showers at camp store, flush toilets, boat ramp, boat rentals, swimming beach

PARKING: At each site

FEE: $16 weekends, $15 weekdays, pack-in sites free but must register

ELEVATION: 847 feet

RESTRICTIONS: *Pets:* On leash only *Fires:* In fire ring *Alcohol:* Prohibited *Vehicles:* 2 per site; no parking on grass *Other:* Quiet hours 10 p.m.–8 a.m.; no visitors after 10 p.m.; gathering firewood prohibited; limit 6 persons per site

desk looking for an open site, not a pack-in site as with some park systems. A mix of sun and shade covers the north campground, and because it lies along a creek bottom, summer camping there may be warmer than at the higher south campground. On the opposite side of the creek, another bridge leads to three rent-a-camps and five additional creek sites, although these creek sites are small with no space for a large tent. Back on the main lane, another small bridge is on the right and leads to the group camping area. A hiking trail is accessible at the forest edge behind the group camp's central fire ring. This hiking trail leads to the south campground and is a leg of the park's nature-filled Ruffed Grouse Trail (0.6 mile). A footpath provides easy walking from the eastern edge of the north campground to the camp store and shower house.

To access the south campground, leave the north campground's entrance and go north on Cutler Lake Road 0.1 mile to Corns Road on the left. Take Corns Road 0.15 mile to the campground entrance on the left. After passing the information station also on the left, sites 1–7 are on the right. These are walk-in sites and offer no view of the lake. Farther up the lane on the left are sites 9, 10, and 12. These sites are smaller, but each is bordered by pines, providing privacy. As the lane makes the turn at the ridge's edge that overlooks the lake, sites 21–25 have wood decks overlooking the lake. Treetops obstruct a clear view of the lake during leafy months, but autumn brings spectacular displays. These five sites require a small tent, as the sites are not big. The nearest sites to the ridge's edge, sites 26–29, offer plenty of tent-pitching space. These sites are also a short walk to the restroom and the Ground Cedar Trail (0.4 mile), which leads to the 0.5-mile-long Vista Trail.

At the opposite end of the lake is a pack-in campground that is reached by walking 0.4 mile from a parking lot on Cutler Lake Road, 0.4 mile east of the camp store. From the parking lot, walk across the road bridge and past the first mowed path on the right. Continue on the road for 50 yards to a second mowed path and signage pointing the way to the pack-in sites and the Ruffed Grouse Nature Trail. The trail is all uphill, but the tranquil setting of the two-site campground is worth

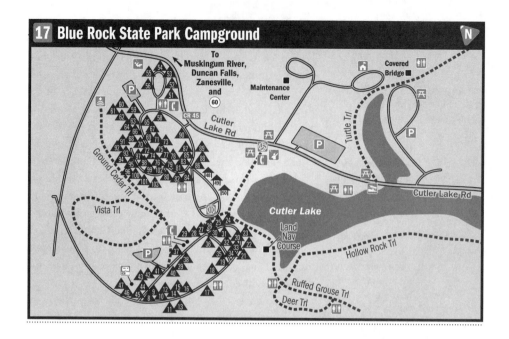

To Muskingum River, Duncan Falls, Zanesville, and 60

Maintenance Center

Covered Bridge

CR 45 Cutler Lake Rd

Turtle Trl

Ground Cedar Trl

Vista Trl

Cutler Lake

Cutler Lake Rd

Land Nav Course

Hollow Rock Trl

Ruffed Grouse Trl

Deer Trl

the effort to get there. A pit latrine, picnic table, and fire rings await those campers looking for a backpacking-type experience. Blue Rock State Forest surrounds the state park with 4,573 acres for exploring. Hiking and equestrian trails roam the creek bottoms and the steep forested hills flanking the waterways. Wildflowers such as trilliums and cardinal flowers, as well as interesting looking mosses and ferns, have a strong presence in and around the forests. Following the Hollow Rock Trail (0.8 mile), which parallels the southern shoreline of Cutler Lake, leads to photographic views of the lake and an abundance of songbirds flittering about and various butterfly species by the thousands.

GETTING THERE

From I-70 Exit 155 in Zanesville, take OH 60 south 10.6 miles through Duncan Falls to Cutler Lake Road on the left. Follow Cutler Lake Road 5.3 miles to Blue Rock State Park.

GPS COORDINATES

N39°49.045'
W81°50.871'

18
BURR OAK COVE

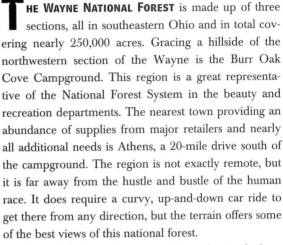

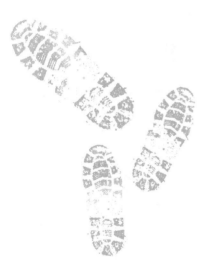

Burr Oak Cove is a highlight of camping in the Wayne National Forest.

THE **WAYNE NATIONAL FOREST** is made up of three sections, all in southeastern Ohio and in total covering nearly 250,000 acres. Gracing a hillside of the northwestern section of the Wayne is the Burr Oak Cove Campground. This region is a great representative of the National Forest System in the beauty and recreation departments. The nearest town providing an abundance of supplies from major retailers and nearly all additional needs is Athens, a 20-mile drive south of the campground. The region is not exactly remote, but it is far away from the hustle and bustle of the human race. It does require a curvy, up-and-down car ride to get there from any direction, but the terrain offers some of the best views of this national forest.

Burr Oak Cove Campground is only 1 mile from the entrance to Burr Oak State Park's campground. The entrance to Burr Oak Cove Campground is identified by the sign that reads WAYNE NATIONAL FOREST CAMPGROUND. The paved campground road quickly leads you to a self-service pay station. Campers have 30 minutes to return to the station and make the correct payment after selecting their site. The towering trees create a canopy over most of the campground, which provides cooler camping in the summer months and an impressive leaf-changing display in the autumn. The 19 sites here are divided along each side of the campground road that leads downhill after passing the pay station. Following the road downhill, the sites on the right side of the road have a brushy backdrop, while the sites on the left have a wooded ravine to their back sides.

The right side–sites have ample tent-pitching room for an extra tent or large cabin tent. During spring and summer, various species of songbirds flittering about the brushy forest's edge and tree limbs emit pleasant audio from early morning well into the evening. The campground remains quiet enough for the birds' performances

RATINGS

Beauty: ☆ ☆ ☆
Privacy: ☆ ☆ ☆
Spaciousness: ☆ ☆ ☆
Quiet: ☆ ☆ ☆ ☆
Security: ☆ ☆
Cleanliness: ☆ ☆

to be heard without interruption. A wide cul-de-sac at the bottom of the hill has its perimeter surrounded with sites. These are spread out well to prevent close neighbors. Going back up the campground road, site 8 will be on the right. This site has a tight parking space, but the camping point of the site is 20 yards from the road, underneath the limbs of towering pines. A wildflower-covered ravine edge (during growing months) skirts two edges of the site. Across the campground road from the pay station is site 2, an ADA-accessible site. This site has a paved walkway leading to a pit latrine. The site is level and the parking space is wide to accommodate a vehicle with a wheelchair lift. Being situated on top of a ridge and near Burr Oak Road, this site gets some light traffic noise.

Two major hiking trails, the North Country Trail and the Buckeye Trail, pass nearby, and it's common to meet thru-hikers at the campground. A joining trail leads from the campground to the Lake View trail, which winds from the dam to the marina of Burr Oak Lake. Several additional hiking trails that lead throughout Burr Oak State Park are only a few minutes' drive away. Paddlers will find striking lake views on the 10-horsepower limit, 644-acre Burr Oak Lake. From Burr Oak Cove Campground, follow Burr Oak Road to CR 63 on the right to find the marina and dock 4. This section of the Wayne National Forest is intersected with well-paved roads that put road touring enthusiasts in position for picturesque views of the lake and surrounding forest.

KEY INFORMATION

ADDRESS:	Wayne National Forest HQ 13700 US 33 Nelsonville, OH 45764
OPERATED BY:	USDA Forest Service, Athens Ranger District
INFORMATION:	(740) 753-0101; www.fs.fed.us/recreation
RESERVATIONS:	None taken
OPEN:	May 15–Sept. 30 with water, year-round without water
SITES:	19; 1 site is ADA accessible
EACH SITE:	Picnic table, fire ring
ASSIGNMENT:	First come, first served
REGISTRATION:	At self-service pay station at entrance
FACILITIES:	Pit latrines, drinking water
PARKING:	At each site
FEE:	$13 per night, $10 per night in winter
ELEVATION:	875 feet
RESTRICTIONS:	*Pets:* On leash and must clean up after *Fires:* In fire ring *Alcohol:* Permitted *Vehicles:* Paved pad for one *Other:* Gathering dead wood from ground is permitted; quiet hours 10 p.m.–6 a.m.; no holding sites for guests arriving later; operation of ATV in campground is prohibited; discharging firearms or fireworks prohibited

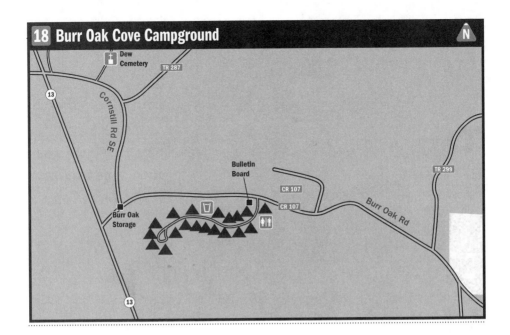

Dew Cemetery

TR 287

13

Cornstill Rd SE

Bulletin Board

CR 107

CR 107

TR 299

Burr Oak Rd

Burr Oak Storage

13

GETTING THERE

From Glouster, take OH 13 north 4.46 miles to Burr Oak Road (CR 107) on the right. Follow Burr Oak Road 0.41 mile to campground entrance on the right.

GPS COORDINATES

N39°33.071'
W82°3.417'

BURR OAK
STATE PARK

THE RIDGES AND HOLLOWS surrounding Burr Oak State Park are foothills of the Appalachian Mountains. A good portion of the natural attractions of the Appalachians can be found and admired at Burr Oak. Nature enthusiasts should visit in spring and fall for hiking or paddling across the 664-acre lake (10-hp limit) to take advantage of the stunning foliage displays. The woodland wildflower displays found along trails and roadsides call for shutterbugs to pause and shoot away. As you drive around the park, keep the windows down to allow the forest environment to please other senses in addition to visual pleasures.

At the camp store on Burr Oak Road, current camping and trail-use information is posted on a bulletin board on the store's porch if the store is closed. Back on Burr Oak Road, travel toward the main campground, and soon after passing the equestrian camp on the left, watch for the Burr Oak water reservoir tower on the right. Near the water tower service driveway is a wooden sign labeled with numbers 82–90. These campsites are not visible right away, but after driving up the service driveway to a small stone parking area, you'll see the camping area situated along the ridge. These nine sites are the most secluded tent sites in the park and require a short walk (approximately 60 feet) to reach them, but the effort is well worth the privacy gained away from the road. The slightly sloping sites are spread out on a finger ridge covered with a mix of hardwood trees and flank both sides of the trail leading through this section. The trail is a portion of a designated park trail marked with blue blazes. This section is often used by backpackers traveling around and through the park. A water spigot is found near the water tower parking lot. But there are no toilets here—you must drive farther down Burr Oak Road 0.62 mile to the main campground bathhouse or go back to the equestrian camp.

A touch of wilderness with plenty of trails to explore it all

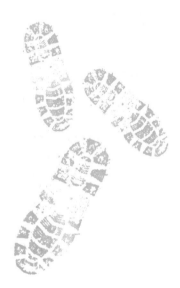

RATINGS

Beauty: ✿ ✿ ✿
Privacy: ✿ ✿ ✿
Spaciousness: ✿ ✿
Quiet: ✿ ✿
Security: ✿ ✿ ✿
Cleanliness: ✿ ✿ ✿

ADDRESS: 10220 Burr Oak
Lodge Road
Glouster, OH 45732

OPERATED BY: ODNR Division of
Parks

INFORMATION: (740) 767-3797;
www.dnr.state
.oh.us/parks

RESERVATIONS: (866) 644-6727;
www.ohio.reserve
world.com

OPEN: Year-round; camp
store/heated show-
ers closed Decem-
ber–March

SITES: 95; 17 with electric,
26 tent only

EACH SITE: Picnic table,
fire ring

ASSIGNMENT: Reservable sites;
walk-in sites first
come, first served

REGISTRATION: At camp store; self-
registration station
on front of store

FACILITIES: Camp store,
showers, flush
toilets, laundry,
payphone, play-
ground, sports
courts, boat ramp,
boat rentals

PARKING: At each site except
for sites 82–90
(designated
parking area)

FEE: $23 electric,
$19 nonelectric

ELEVATION: 896 feet

RESTRICTIONS: *Pets:* At all sites—on
leash only
Fires: In fire ring
Alcohol: Prohibited
Vehicles: 1 per site
Other: Quiet hours
10 p.m.–8 a.m.;
gathering firewood
prohibited; 14-day
stay limit

The main campground is located on a peninsula. Burr Oak Road ends at a cul-de-sac surrounded by sites 12–29. Ten of those sites overlook the lake, but they don't allow much space for large tents or direct access to the lake. The drop-off from sites 18–24 to the lake's edge is separated by safety netting to keep young campers from falling over the ledge. Sites 1–11 and 30–60 are suited for RVs and are a bit close to the neighboring sites. Sites 65–81 are tent-only. These tent sites skirt a ridge edge—all 16 sites are situated on a shelf cut into a hillside. A few of these sites are tough to maneuver from vehicle to site setup, as the slope from the parking space to the site is steep. Site 67 is the best of these tent sites because it provides the largest level area for a tent and a drinking water spigot is nearby. Several boat docks serve the sprawling lake, and two of them have campsites—docks 2 and 3. Dock 2 has 13 sites, and dock 3 has 8 primitive sites.

The rugged geography of the park attracts many hikers and backpackers seeking the challenging trails. Included in the park's hiking trails are 28 miles of the state's Buckeye Trail and North Country Trail. The Wildcat Hollow Backpack Trail is a star attraction and legitimate backpacking trail, offering enough adventure for two days of exploration. This 14.7-mile loop's trailhead is located on Burr Oak Lodge Road, off OH 78, which branches east off OH 13 just north of Glouster. The 1-mile Campground Trail runs from the equestrian camp to the main campground, with most of the trail overlooking the lake.

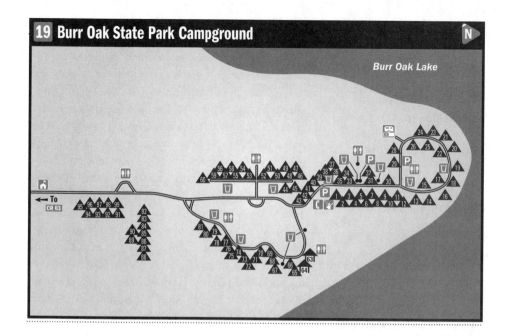

Burr Oak Lake

GETTING THERE

From Glouster, take OH 13 north 4.46 miles to Burr Oak Road (CR 107) on the right. Follow Burr Oak Road 1.53 miles to the first campsites on the right; then continue on Burr Oak Road 0.31 mile to reach the main campground area.

GPS COORDINATES

N39°32.572'
W82°2.391'

20
COVERED BRIDGE
SCENIC BYWAY

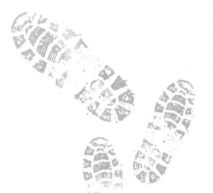

One beautiful byway features five appealing campgrounds.

THE **COVERED BRIDGE SCENIC BYWAY** (CBSB) is a 44-mile tour through southeastern Ohio. The designated scenic stretch of winding and rolling State Route 26 runs from Marietta to Woodsfield—cutting through a mix of agriculture and forest landscapes. The covered bridges that remain from the horse and buggy days of the 1800s stand proud and welcome the attention of admirers. Along this driving tour you will see a variety of vehicle types cruising the pavement, with the operators and passengers enthralled with the scenery. This stretch of road also cuts through a portion of the Wayne National Forest, which adds a touch of wild country to the trip. Wandering alongside the CBSB for many of the 44 miles is the Little Muskingum River, a pleasant little river that hosts paddlers nearly year-round. For the most part, the river's water slowly finds its way to the Muskingum River, which dumps into the Ohio River at Marietta. Spotted along the Little Muskingum River and the CBSB are five small campgrounds, with each one offering its own flavor to satisfy campers of varying camping appetites.

RATINGS

LANE FARM CAMPGROUND
Beauty: ✿ ✿
Privacy: ✿
Spaciousness: ✿ ✿
Quiet: ✿
Security: ✿ ✿
Cleanliness: ✿

HUNE BRIDGE CAMPGROUND
Beauty: ✿ ✿
Privacy: ✿
Spaciousness: ✿ ✿
Quiet: ✿ ✿
Security: ✿ ✿
Cleanliness: ✿

HAUGHT RUN CAMPGROUND
Beauty: ✿ ✿
Privacy: ✿ ✿
Spaciousness: ✿ ✿
Quiet: ✿ ✿ ✿
Security: ✿ ✿
Cleanliness: ✿ ✿

RING MILL CAMPGROUND
Beauty: ✿ ✿
Privacy: ✿ ✿
Spaciousness: ✿ ✿
Quiet: ✿ ✿ ✿
Security: ✿
Cleanliness: ✿ ✿

LAMPING HOMESTEAD CAMPGROUND
Beauty: ✿ ✿ ✿
Privacy: ✿ ✿ ✿
Spaciousness: ✿ ✿
Quiet: ✿ ✿ ✿ ✿
Security: ✿
Cleanliness: ✿ ✿

ADDRESS: Marietta Unit, Athens Ranger District
27750 State Route 7
Marietta, OH 45750

OPERATED BY: USDA Forest Service, Athens Ranger District, Marietta Unit

INFORMATION: (740) 373-9055; www.fs.fed.us/recreation

RESERVATIONS: First-come, first-served basis

OPEN: Year-round

SITES: Lane Farm Campground: 4; Hune Bridge Campground: 3; Haught Run Campground: 4; Ring Mill Campground: 3; Lamping Homestead Campground: 6

EACH SITE: Picnic table, fire ring

ASSIGNMENT: First come, first served

REGISTRATION: No registration

FACILITIES: Pit latrine

PARKING: At each site (except Lamping Homestead Campground has parking area)

FEE: Free

ELEVATION: Lane Farm Campground: 612 feet; Hune Bridge Campground: 637 feet; Haught Run Campground: 669 feet; Ring Mill Campground: 679 feet; Lamping Homestead Campground: 734 feet

RESTRICTIONS: *Pets:* Must be kept on leash and cleaned up after
Fires: In fire ring
Alcohol: Permitted
Vehicles: Multiple allowed
Other: Gathering dead wood from ground for firewood is permitted; quiet hours 10 p.m.–6 a.m.; no holding sites for guests arriving later; operation of ATV in campground is prohibited; discharging firearms or fireworks prohibited; 14-day stay limit; most supplies found in Marietta and Woodsfield

For tent campers, the campgrounds seem to improve as you travel northeast on the CBSB, beginning in Marietta. The first is the Lane Farm Campground, 5.05 miles from Marietta. The four sites perched on a high bank of the Little Muskingum are visited more than those farther down the road because of their closeness to town. This campground is just off of SR 26, and road noise is a constant presence. A canoe launching–area is temporarily closed as the steps leading down the steep riverbank were washed out by winter ice. Agile canoers might still maneuver their watercrafts to the water at a point near site 1. Sites 1 and 2 offer the best shade for summer camping and are the most spacious, if friends are along for the river excursion. A unisex pit latrine is located a short walk from the sites, but not too close. The North Country Trail drops into camp here from the opposite side of the river. When the river is at average water levels it can be crossed here with caution—but hold packs up high.

Driving northeast on Route 26 for 12.1 miles from Lane Farm Campground, you will see the Hune Bridge on the right. Cross the bridge to find the Hune Bridge Campground on the bridge's south side. Three sites are spaced well apart, with the last sitting near the river. The Little Muskingum River at this point is wide with a broad strip of gravel riverbank to explore or drop a line to catch your dinner. The easy access to the river here means this area is also utilized as a canoe loading and pulling site. From the campground you can

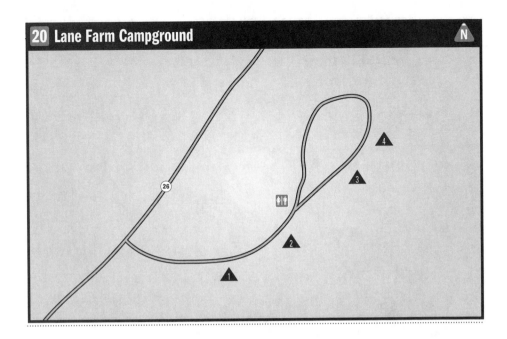

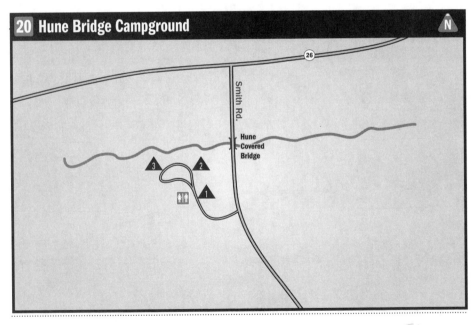

access a 5-mile-long hiking trail to Haught Run Campground, which lies to the northeast and is the next stop along the CBSB. There are two interpretive signs at the Hune camp. The first provides historical information regarding the bridge, and the other explains the importance of the oil and gas industry of today in the region. An oil-gathering tank, complete with lines slithering out of it and into the forest, is on display at the campground.

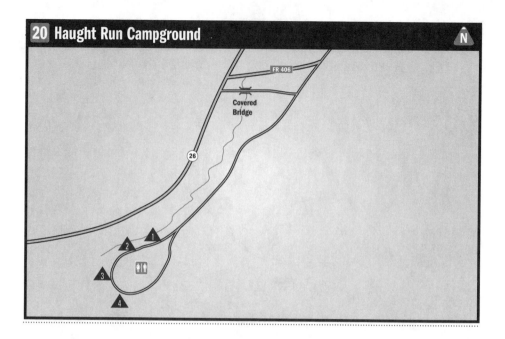

Covered
Bridge

26

FR 406

1
2
3
4

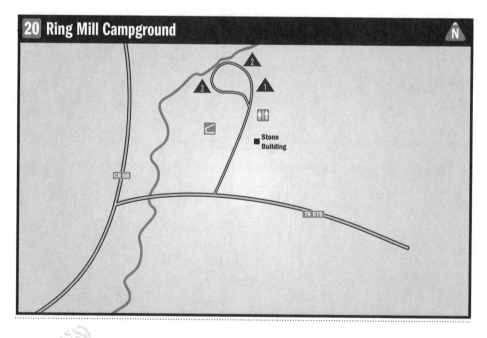

2
3
1

Stone
Building

CR 68

TR 575

Back on Route 26, and 3.58 miles farther, you will arrive at the Rinard Bridge and access to the Haught Run Campground. The bridge comes into view on the right, but you won't see the campground there. After turning right onto the modern bridge just north of the covered bridge, take another right after making the crossing onto a gravel road. Follow the gravel road 0.47 mile to the pleasant little campground situated in a wood grove that provides privacy from Route 26 (not far from the opposing riverbank). The four well-spaced sites here have newly paved parking pads and stone fire rings. A maintained latrine exists, but there is no drinking water here, just as with the other four CBSB campgrounds. This point of the Little Muskingum River might offer the best fishing, with several deeper runs and submerged fish-holding habitat. Fly fishers are known to frequent this campground and spend a couple days casting a few flies here in hopes of catching smallmouth bass. While driving the gravel access road to the campground, keep an eye on the river paralleling the road and you may catch a glimpse of raccoons and minks doing some fishing as well.

The next campground is not within eye- or earshot of Route 26. From the Rinard Bridge, follow Route 26 for 10.77 miles to CR 68 on the right. Drive 2.70 miles to TR 575 on the right, cross the bridge over the Little Muskingum, and the Ring Mill Campground lane is on the left. After entering the lane, you will see an old stone building on the right. An interpretive sign next to the road tells the story of the building's history as the home of the family than ran a mill on the site during the mid 1800s (listed on the National Register of Historic Places). Take a moment here to imagine what life was like at this place 150 years ago. Continue down the lane to three campsites and a new shelter house, with a latrine located near the stone building. Site 3 is on the river, and sites 1 and 2 are farther back. Direct access to the river from site 3 is difficult as the bank is steep, but there is a canoe access lane adjacent to the site. The campground is mostly shaded except for the open canopy bordering the lane. This campground may be the least visited of the five CBSB campgrounds. This campground is also a trailhead for the North Country Trail and Ohio's statewide hiking trail, the Buckeye Trail.

Return to Route 26 and drive 2.85 miles to OH 537 on the left. Follow this road for 1.64 miles up and around a tall ridge that gives a great view of the valley you just came through, before descending down the back side of the ridge to Clearfork Road on the left. Go 0.14 mile to the Lamping Homestead Campground—one of Ohio's best tent camping opportunities. Park your car in the gravel parking area and look toward the large pond beyond the mowed field. The six sites (and picnic shelter) are tucked under the towering pines on the pond's edge on your left—you have to walk approximately 60 yards from the parking area to the campsites. The field is level, which makes it easy to traverse. A latrine is located near the parking area, where you can also find a bulletin board with information including advice for keeping food stored to deter black bear visits.

The sites here are equally level and pleasantly situated with views of the pond. The 2-acre pond is stocked with bass, bluegill, and catfish, so pack a rod and reel. The setting here in the autumn is a must-photograph scene. Even if all six sites are occupied, there is plenty of space for every camper to experience the remote, wild essence felt here. Two hiking trails loop out into the forest from the campground. One is 1.5 miles long, and the other is a 3.5-mile trek with several views from the surrounding ridges. A cemetery rests on a hill above the campground that holds some of the Lamping family members. The Lampings settled on the property in the early 1800s before sickness and hard living forced the remaining family members to move on. What exists on the site today is a retreat from today's trials and tribulations.

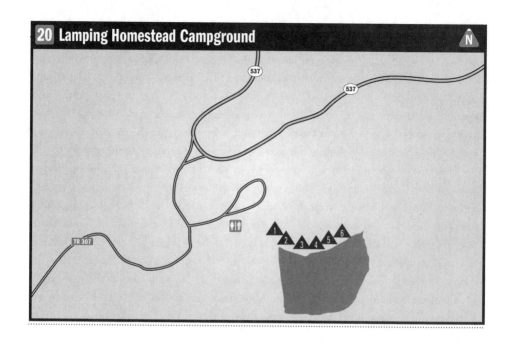

GETTING THERE

Take Exit 1 from I-77 at Marietta. Go west on OH 7 and turn right onto Acme Street (first traffic light). Drive 0.63 mile to Greene Street (OH 26) then turn right. Travel 5.05 miles to Lane Farm Campground on right.

GPS COORDINATES

LANE FARM CAMPGROUND:
N39°26.145'
W81°21.553'

HUNE BRIDGE CAMPGROUND:
N39°30.573'
W81°15.014'

HAUGHT RUN CAMPGROUND:
N39°31.934'
W81°13.492'

RING MILL CAMPGROUND:
N39°36.445'
W81°7.320'

LAMPING HOMESTEAD CAMPGROUND:
N39°37.823'
W81°11.423'

21
FORKED RUN
STATE PARK

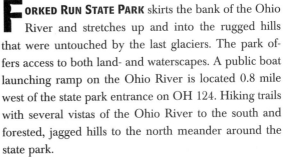

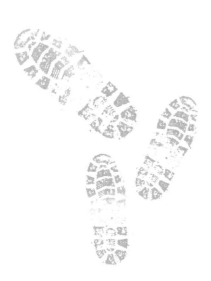

Rugged forest country overlooking the Ohio River

FORKED RUN STATE PARK skirts the bank of the Ohio River and stretches up and into the rugged hills that were untouched by the last glaciers. The park offers access to both land- and waterscapes. A public boat launching ramp on the Ohio River is located 0.8 mile west of the state park entrance on OH 124. Hiking trails with several vistas of the Ohio River to the south and forested, jagged hills to the north meander around the state park.

Just as folks did a century or more ago, today's campers set up on a ridgetop high above the Ohio River and enjoy views of both the grand river and dense forest covering the crest. The campground consists of five sections set on top of three sharp hills. Area One (sites 1–52) attracts RVers on a regular basis because of the amenities close by. A heated-shower house sits in the center of Area One, with the amphitheater, playground, and rental cabins along the road here. Area One is found by taking the first left after passing by the campground office, atop the shortest of the three mini-mountains.

Area Two (sites 53–76) is on the next left once back on the main campground road, ascending the second hill. Area Two's 23 sites offer electricity but a primitive feel. The sites are spaced out enough to give a bit of privacy, and during the week you may hardly see another person in this section. Site 67 sits at the top of this hill, at the outer edge of the cul de sac, facing west. During autumn, site 67 puts leaf peepers in a front row seat to a fall season sunset over the Ohio River.

Continue around the main campground road from Area Two, and a shower house sits at a crossroads. Turn left to access Area Three. Area Three's (sites 77–122) sites are sprinkled along both sides of a snaking 0.68-mile incline to the highest peak—200 feet in elevation gain from the park entrance—before reaching a small

RATINGS

Beauty: ☆ ☆
Privacy: ☆ ☆
Spaciousness: ☆ ☆
Quiet: ☆ ☆
Security: ☆ ☆
Cleanliness: ☆ ☆ ☆

loop. Halfway up the road on the left are sites 118 and 119—each makes a pleasant place to tent camp, on a shelf cut along the ridge's back, and includes a view to the west, across a ravine and to a neighboring hilltop. At the top and the loop, site 100 sits next to a water spigot facing the west for a sunset display at day's end. Near site 100 are two trailheads. The first is the 2.6-mile Lakeview Trail which, true to its name, delivers a rigorous trek down the ridge within view of the lake. The trail continues around the side of the hill and arrives at the sandy swimming beach before turning and traversing the hill toward campground Area Three. The second trail is the 0.75-mile Riverview Trail, which leads to a scenic look at the Ohio River coursing below.

Back to the intersection of campground roads, the small Area Four (sites 123–130) is on the left. This nonelectric section is small for anything larger than a four-person dome tent. The parking spaces are at the road's edge and the campsites can be reached by taking a few steps down a slope to a small landing at the wood's edge. Return to the campground road; turn left and follow it to Area Five (sites 131–151). This is the closet area to the 120-acre Forked Run Lake, which offers respectable crappie fishing. It is tough to fish from the shore here, however, as the steep hills plunge straight into the lake. Because this park is well off of the beaten path, the lake receives few boaters, making it perfectly suited for kayak fishing. Area Five's 20 sites sit dotted along a sparsely shaded ridge. Most of these sites are well spaced and can accommodate a family-sized tent.

The 2,475-acre Shade River State Forest joins this state park to the north. A short drive through the state forest via township roads reveals current forest management practices in action.

KEY INFORMATION

ADDRESS: P.O. Box 127 Reedsville, OH 45772-0127

OPERATED BY: ODNR Division of Parks

INFORMATION: (740) 378-6206; www.dnr.state .oh.us/parks

RESERVATIONS: (866) 644-6727; www.ohio.reserve world.com

OPEN: Year-round; heated showers and camp store closed December–March

SITES: 64 nonelectric; 81 electric

EACH SITE: Picnic table, fire ring

ASSIGNMENT: Reservable sites; walk-in sites first come, first served

REGISTRATION: Self-registration station at campground office if office is closed

FACILITIES: Showers, vault latrines, laundry, camp store, sports courts, playground, swimming beach, boat rentals, disc golf course

PARKING: At each site

FEE: $19 nonelectric; $23 electric; $2 off in winter; $1 off Sunday–Thursday regular season

ELEVATION: 649 feet

RESTRICTIONS: *Pets:* On leash only *Fires:* In fire ring *Alcohol:* Prohibited *Vehicles:* 1 per site *Other:* Quiet hours 10 p.m.–8 a.m.; gathering firewood prohibited; limit 6 persons per site

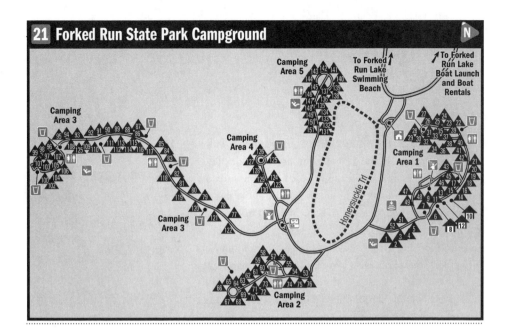

GETTING THERE

From Pomeroy, follow OH 7 east for 6.07 miles to Chester. Take OH 248 east for 9.03 miles to OH 124. Turn left and travel east for 1.85 miles to the park entrance on the left.

GPS COORDINATES

N39°5.503'
W81°46.335'

THE MATURE DECIDUOUS TREES of Hocking Hills perform one of the best autumn leaf color displays in the state. For this reason, the park has thousands of fall visitors at the campgrounds and cruising the park's roadways and hiking trails. If you had to choose one camping experience from this book for the fall foliage season, Hocking Hills would be it. This area's natural attractions include caves, gorges, and the abundance of access to these natural wonders by well-maintained hiking trails and surrounding county and state roads. The park's caves can be accessed by even physically challenged outdoors enthusiasts. One of the most popular caves, Ash Cave, is accessed from a paved parking area with bathrooms via a level, paved walking trail. Old Man's Cave, the most visited cave of the park, is near the main campground entrance. There are several parks within a few minutes' drive of Old Man's Cave, so expect to go back again and again to explore more picturesque stone formations. For rock climbers, a designated area on Big Pine Road off of OH 374 in the Hocking Hills State Forest, offers 100-foot cliffs, chimneys, and overhangs to get a hands-on feel for the scenic Hocking Hills.

Hocking Hills State Park runs one of the most popular family campgrounds in the state, which means that Old Man's Cave Family Campground is buzzing on a regular basis. It includes 156 electric sites that draw their fair share of RVers. To avoid the bustling campground with campers milling about like an active anthill, another Hocking Hills family campground offers some relief. The Family Primitive Hike-In Camp is less than a mile away from the primary campground entrance. From the primary campground office on OH 664—where all campsites are paid for and registered—travel north for 0.53 mile to OH 374. The next left leads to the hike-in campground parking area.

> *Caves, gorges, and waterfalls pepper southern Ohio's premier hiking destination.*

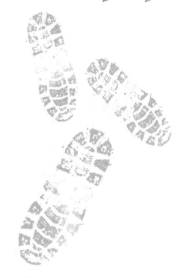

RATINGS

Beauty: ✩ ✩ ✩
Privacy: ✩ ✩ ✩
Spaciousness: ✩ ✩ ✩
Quiet: ✩ ✩ ✩
Security: ✩ ✩
Cleanliness: ✩ ✩

ADDRESS:	19852 SR 664 Logan, OH 43138-9537
OPERATED BY:	ODNR Division of State Parks
INFORMATION:	(740) 385-6841; www.dnr.state .oh.us/parks
RESERVATIONS:	(866) 644-6727; www.ohio.reserve world.com
OPEN:	April 1–November 15; Old Man's Cave Campground year-round
SITES:	33 Family Hike-In Area; 13 nonelectric; 156 electric at main campground
EACH SITE:	Fire ring
ASSIGNMENT:	Reservable sites; walk-in sites first come, first served
REGISTRATION:	At office at main campground entrance on OH 664
FACILITIES:	Family Hike-In Area: latrines, water supply; main campground: showers, flush toilets, laundry, camp store, pool
PARKING:	In gravel lot
FEE:	$21; $1 off Sun.– Thurs.; $2 off in winter
ELEVATION:	1,020 feet
RESTRICTIONS:	*Pets:* On leash only *Fires:* In fire ring *Alcohol:* Prohibited *Vehicles:* No vehicles permitted in Family Hike-In Area *Other:* Quiet hours 10 p.m.–8 a.m.; gathering firewood prohibited; limit 6 persons per site

The parking area is adjacent to the park's maintenance shop, with a water spigot for use by campers between the parking area and the shop. The 33 tent sites here can be accessed only on foot. The campground lane extends more than a half mile into the forest, rolling and alternating left and right only slightly—a moderate walk at best is all that is needed to reach the most remote site. All sites are situated along the road, some only a step away from the forest road's edge and others a dozen or so yards to the left or right of the road. The distance from the parking area to the first site is only 20 yards, but to reach the last site at the end of the road, a 0.6-mile hike is required. Watch out for the occasional mountain biker, as the 2-mile Purple Trail uses the campground road as a leg of the course.

Sites 1–5 are first come, first served; the other 28 sites are reservable. Latrines sit near the first site, a few sites from the road's end. Site 6 is nearly hidden from the road thanks to a 20-yard path, but it does catch some road noise from OH 374 through the forest. Site 8 is down a slope from the road and quieter, as OH 374 turns away from the campground slightly here. Site 9 sits on a mound off to the right, nearly hidden from passersby (unless they are gazing up at the crown of a mix of oaks and hickories). Down the road 30 yards and to the left is site 29, which drops down a slant and curves out of site behind some young trees and heavy brush.

Site 10 is near the road's halfway point—a wide site with ample space for parent tent and kiddie tents. This site is only a step off the road, so expect some "hellos." A narrow path lined with trees leads to site 28, which sits on the sheltered side of the road. Sites 12 and 28 are neighbors with the road between them. These sites work well for sociable campers who don't mind the sounds of footsteps and bike tires passing close by. Site 22 sits at the end of the road, 30 yards from the next-to-last site. It is wide and level, and the most private site here—the reward for hauling all your gear and accepting the fact that if something was left in the car, it would take a 1-mile-plus trek to retrieve it. The difference in the highest and lowest elevation of the campground road is 40 feet.

About a half mile south on OH 374 from the hike-in campground sign is a small parking area on the right.

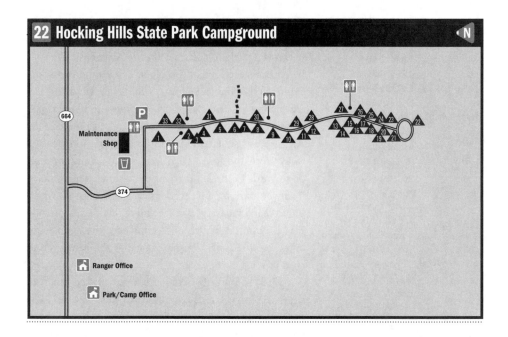

Leave the car and follow the half-mile hiking trail to the remote, 17-acre Rose Lake. The lake is stocked annually with rainbow trout; a wide dam and several spots along the wooded shoreline offer a few casting spots. In the spring, keep a keen eye along the trail for a real treat: edible morel mushrooms that may have just popped from the deciduous leaf clutter on the forest floor.

GETTING THERE

From Logan, travel south on OH 664 for 10.29 miles to OH 374 on the left. Follow OH 374 for 0.33 mile to the park service lane on the left. The Family Primitive Hike-In Area parking is straight ahead.

GPS COORDINATES

N39°26.164'
W82°31.511'

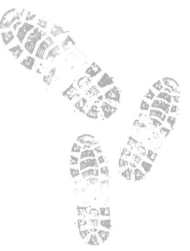

> *This pleasing little park and lake are nestled in the Appalachian Highlands.*

WHAT WAS CREATED to be a private amusement park during the early 1900s is now a naturally amusing destination surrounding the round, 60-acre Lake Alma, which includes an island in the middle for exploring. Lake Alma State Park is not a big park, but what it lacks in size it makes up for in quality. This lake is at its best for paddling and photography in spring and fall. The lake's aquatic diversity decorating the shoreline keeps shutterbugs busy for hours and canoers and kayakers entertained for a full day, and then some. A one-way park road circles the lake and park, with one side designated for walkers and bikers. Be sure to make a loop around the park road and see what this little park has to offer before settling into your campsite.

The primary campground spreads out along the valley floor formed by two hills overlooking the eastern shore of Lake Alma. A small but pleasant camp office offers visitors an abundance of information on current events, and a few supplies. Posted on exterior bulletin boards at the campground office are a series of photos of the park in action beginning nearly a century ago. Approximately 100 feet south of the office on the left is the entrance to the campsites. The first string of eight campsites on the left are often filled with RVs, and the sites across the road from those offer little space for a tent. As you drive farther up the narrow valley, the sites get more appealing.

The next small group of sites on the right is better spaced for a tent spread. Sites 16 and 17 are ideal, as they offer the most room and a fire ring closer to the rear of the site, away from the campground road. As you pass site 20 on the right, turn right and sites 65–73 will be visible lining one side of the paved road leading deep into a branch of the valley. These sites have a deep drainage ditch at their rear, but they offer ample room for setting up a camp (at which you may wish to

RATINGS

Beauty: ✰ ✰
Privacy: ✰ ✰
Spaciousness: ✰ ✰
Quiet: ✰ ✰
Security: ✰ ✰ ✰
Cleanliness: ✰ ✰ ✰

include a portable sun shower, as the campground has no shower facilities). Across the road from this row of sites is the steep, wooded hillside that provides views of wild critters as they scamper about. At the end of the row, sitting alone at the outer edge of the cul de sac, is site 73. To the left of site 73 is space for a minimal campsite set up. To the right of the site is a wider, grassy area. At the rear of that grassy area is a wooden foot bridge that accesses the 0.75-mile Sassafras Trail. This hiking trail climbs north over the southern, forested hill and arrives near the campground entrance.

Travel back to the road intersection near site 20 and stay to the right. A water fountain and pit latrine sit at the intersection, both an easy, 100-foot walk from site 73. The campground continues up the ravine as it narrows, with sites 34–38 at the end of the dead end road. These five sites have trees guarding the corners of the parking spaces, which make backing an RV in nearly impossible. As a result, tent campers should have this quiet end of the campground to themselves. Behind the sites is a small stream for kids to explore. During heavy rain events the stream will fill suddenly because of the steepness of the surrounding hills. But the creek banks are high enough to keep most water contained and out of the campsites. Site 34 is the last site on the road; because there is no place to turn around except for the parking space of site 34, sightseeing vehicles may be unwelcome guests from time to time.

Ten primitive sites sit along Little Raccoon Creek on the opposite side of the lake. Sites 74–83 are found on the west side of OH 349, near the park's entrance. Not all of the sites are marked, but a picnic table and fire ring reveal each site's location. In the same area are a shelter house and basketball court, which brings families close, so privacy and complete solitude are not qualities likely to be had here. Water is available at a drinking fountain at the shelter house, and pit latrines and a portable toilet are there as well.

Five miles to the northwest of the state park is the Leo Petroglyph State Memorial, preserved and protected by the Ohio Historical Society. The petroglyph includes 37 drawings of animals and humans, created by the Fort Ancient Indians more than 500 years ago. The

KEY INFORMATION

ADDRESS:	422 Lake Alma Rd. Wellston, OH 45692
OPERATED BY:	ODNR Division of State Parks
INFORMATION:	(740) 384-4474; www.dnr.state .oh.us/parks
RESERVATIONS:	(866) 644-6727; www.ohio.reserve world.com
OPEN:	Year-round; limited facilities in winter months
SITES:	10 nonelectric; 71 electric
EACH SITE:	Picnic table, fire ring
ASSIGNMENT:	Reservable sites; walk-in sites first come, first served
REGISTRATION:	Self-registration station at campground office, if office closed
FACILITIES:	Pit latrines, water fountains, camp store, sports courts, playground, swimming beach, boat rentals, nature center, pay phone at camp office
PARKING:	At each site
FEE:	$23 electric; $19 nonelectric
ELEVATION:	687 feet
RESTRICTIONS:	*Pets:* On leash only *Fires:* In fire ring *Alcohol:* Prohibited *Vehicles:* 1 per site *Other:* Quiet hours 10 p.m.–8 a.m.; gathering firewood prohibited; limit 6 persons per site

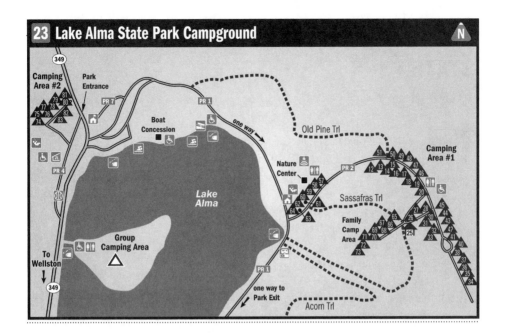

GETTING THERE

From Wellston, go north on OH 93 for 0.7 mile to OH 349. Turn right and travel 1.53 miles to the park entrance on the right. Follow the park road 0.44 mile to the campground entrance on the left.

small park includes an observation deck and a walking trail through the sandstone gorge that provided protection to the Native Americans. To find the memorial and its small parking lot, leave Lake Alma State Park and go south to Wellston. Travel northwest on OH 327 for 6.31 miles to County Road 30 on the left. Follow CR 30 for 2.19 miles to CR 29 and turn left. Travel 0.63 mile to Township Road 224 on the right; follow it 0.46 mile to a parking lot on the left.

GPS COORDINATES

N39°8.786'
W82°30.589'

24
LAKE HOPE
STATE PARK

THE GLACIAL MELTWATERS that carved their way
through southeastern Ohio left behind a rugged
landscape. Thousands of years later, those ravines and
their accompanying ridges are now covered with forests
and interspersed meadows offering nature lovers a paradise to explore. When visiting the Lake Hope State Park
region, bring either a pair of sturdy hiking boots and/or
a trusted mountain bike because the park presents more
than 23 miles of trails for both. While driving to and
through this state park, it quickly becomes evident that
you are somewhere special. Surrounded by the Zaleski
State Forest, Lake Hope State Park opportunities for
adventure are nearly limitless, including rock climbing,
extreme hiking, serious mountain biking, kayaking, and
horseback riding on what may be the most beautiful
equine trail in the state. A wildflower guidebook will
also be useful while visiting Zaleski as the forest is home
to numerous species, such as blue-eyed Mary and the
wild geranium. The 120-acre Lake Hope is impressive
in its own right, perfect for kayaking or canoeing, or
simply sitting at its edge and dangling a toe into the
crystal-clear water.

This pleasant campground sees many repeat campers for several reasons, primarily the abundance of
outdoor pursuits available and the gorgeous scenery.
Campground sites are staged along a 2-mile-long ridge
covered with a mix of deciduous and evergreen forests
and views overlooking deep valleys and ridgetops.

After passing the nature center and then the campground office, walk-in sites 1–28 and 177–190 are first
come, first served. As the ridge continues to rise and you
travel on, sites 33–35 require a short, steep walk downhill from their parking spaces. Those sites are perched
on a ledge with limited views of the next ridge. During
the fall, these ridges seem to glow orange and bright red
for miles with the transforming leaves. The main shower

> *Tent camping is a treat at
> Lake Hope State Park.*

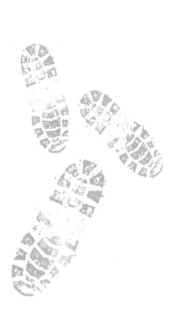

RATINGS

Beauty: ✩ ✩
Privacy: ✩ ✩ ✩
Spaciousness: ✩ ✩ ✩
Quiet: ✩ ✩ ✩
Security: ✩ ✩ ✩ ✩
Cleanliness: ✩ ✩ ✩

ADDRESS:	27331 SR 278 McArthur, OH 45651
OPERATED BY:	ODNR Division of Parks
INFORMATION:	(740) 596-5253; www.dnr.state .oh.us/parks
RESERVATIONS:	(866) 644-6727; www.ohio.reserve world.com
OPEN:	Year-round (sites 1–28 and 177–192); April–December (sites 29–89); April–September (sites 90–125)
SITES:	141 nonelectric; 46 electric
EACH SITE:	Picnic table, fire ring
ASSIGNMENT:	Reservable sites; walk-in sites first come, first served
REGISTRATION:	At campground office; self-register if office closed
FACILITIES:	Showers, latrines, laundry, pay phone, nature center, playground, sports courts, boat ramp, boat rentals at Lake Hope
PARKING:	At each site
FEE:	$22 electric; $18 nonelectric; $2 off fee in winter
ELEVATION:	919 feet
RESTRICTIONS:	*Pets:* On leash only *Fires:* In fire ring *Alcohol:* Prohibited *Vehicles:* 1 per site; additional parking available *Other:* Quiet hours 10 p.m.–8 a.m.; gathering firewood prohibited

house is located near sites 62–89, with a second shower house near the camp office. Those sites have electricity and are usually taken by RVers. Leave the shower house site and continue through a gate that is closed during winter months. After passing through the gate, tent campers should feel more at home in sites 90–125, which grace the top of a smaller finger ridge. This section of the campground features large pines and a steady breeze, so be sure those tent stakes are well placed. This section has the feel of a western mountain forest campground, with the wind whispering through the pine branches and the aroma of pine needles. Sites 100–108 are suited for smaller tents and tent campers with very little gear. Sites 109 and 114 are small group sites. The Habron Hollow hiking trail can be accessed from site 114. The trail rolls down the ridge for more than 1.5 miles where another hiking trail, the White Oak hiking trail comes in from the left. Follow this adjoining trail for a nice 0.25-mile trek to the camp office. Two mountain bike trails split off from the Habron Hollow trail: the Red Oak Bike Trail, which leads back to the campground's main road, and the 7.2-mile Copperhead Bike Trail.

A first-class nature center draws its share of visitors of all ages to interact with naturalists and explore the many displays. In July and August, feeding hummingbirds by hand is a popular pastime. Some interesting remnants of the area's past include the iron furnaces that were once a bustling industry here. The Hope Furnace was used more than 100 years ago to process the iron ore taken from the region's sandstone. The iron was then used for items such as ammunition cannons for the Union Army during the Civil War. The charcoal fires that burned 24 hours a day used a great quantity of wood from area woodlands, until the iron smelting ceased here around 1900. Today, the forests have been replenished, and the Hope Furnace chimney and a portion of the foundation remain near the campground entrance.

Note: Visitors must register at the park office on OH 278. Major retailers are in Nelsonville.

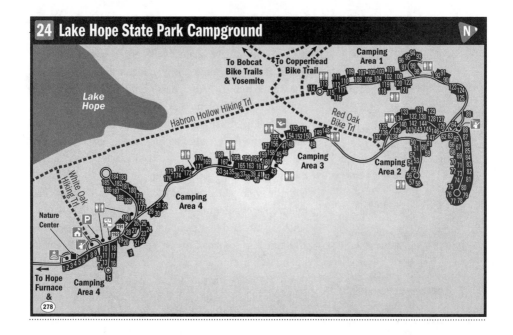

GETTING THERE

From OH 33 in Nelsonville, take OH 278 south 12.77 miles to Furnace Ridge Road on the right. Travel up a steep, windy road 0.56 mile to the campground office.

GPS COORDINATES

N39°20.147'
W82°20.430'

One of Ohio's premium tent-camping destinations

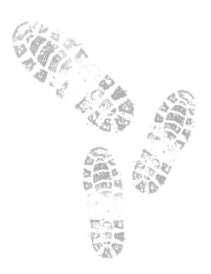

GAZING OUT OVER the dense forest of the Wayne National Forest at the Lake Vesuvius Recreation Area today, one can hardly imagine the hills bare of trees. This was the case in the early 1900s, however, due to extensive timber harvesting to fuel the area's iron ore furnaces, which were active in the 1800s. What is visible today are the results of years of hard work initiated by the Civilian Conservation Corp during the 1930s, and the recreational opportunities created by forest managers over the last several decades. There are more than 1,200 acres of big woods to explore here, as well as the 143-acre lake. Healthy hikers can hit the 8-mile Lakeshore Trail that chases the lake's edge, with views of rock outcroppings and footbridge crossings for an up-close look at this section of a national forest. Start that trek at any of the several parking sites around the lake

There are two campgrounds to choose from at Lake Vesuvius. A major renovation of one of those campgrounds in 2010 makes it appealing to RVers, while the other remains a dandy place to escape in a tent. Traveling on CR 29 from OH 93, the first road on the left leads to the updated Oak Hill Campground, consisting of newly paved roads and site pads, new shower and toilet facilities, electricity, and water. Campers staying at the older, but more pleasantly connected-to-nature campground, Iron Ridge Campground, stay across the lake and alone on a forested ridge.

Where the road to Oak Hill Campground turned off of CR 29, continue east on CR 29 and pass below the lake's spillway and historic ore furnace on the right. Continue on to the next road to the left. This dead-end road snakes uphill to Iron Ridge, which has sites on each side of the road all the way to a small loop. The campground stretches out over one-half mile. At the entrance to this ideal woodland camping experience are a self-registration station and bulletin board on the right. To

RATINGS

Beauty: ✿ ✿ ✿ ✿
Privacy: ✿ ✿ ✿
Spaciousness: ✿ ✿ ✿
Quiet: ✿ ✿ ✿ ✿
Security: ✿ ✿ ✿
Cleanliness: ✿ ✿ ✿

the left is the first site, occupied by a campground host. The next seven sites offer electricity and remain attractive to tent campers because of their remoteness.

A dozen yards uphill from site 8 on the left is a small parking area and latrine for sites 9–16, which are walk-in sites. These eight sites populate the top of a finger ridge facing the south. Even with the heavy forest cover, expect some sun to penetrate to warm up camp. It's a 40-yard distance from the parking area to site 16. Each site is staggered down the ridge, giving each site plenty of privacy. The only thing crowded on this ridge, and anywhere in the Iron Ridge Campground, are the trees in this healthy deciduous and evergreen forest.

Nearing the top of the ridge is another set of walk-in sites—sites 26–28. These three sites differ from the first set of walk-in sites as they run parallel to the road and are less than ten yards from the road's edge. From the small parking area, there are no sites until you reach the loop at the end of the road. Inside the loop is a latrine and water spigot. As the loop turns and begins to descend, site 35 sits on the outside with the highest viewpoint from the ridge. Next to this site is the arrival of the Whiskey Run Trail, a half-mile hiking trail connecting the campground to the lake and the Lake Shore Trail, 150 feet below the top of the ridge.

Lake Vesuvius is as picturesque as a big forest lake gets. The lake is accessible by all, thanks to the 0.32-mile-long boardwalk that links the dam and spillway to the south to the boat dock at the northern tip of the lake's western branch. The boardwalk skirts along the shoreline and includes several wide sections for anglers to cast a line without any interference. Beginning at the boat dock parking lot is the 0.75-mile Rock House Trail, an interpretive, paved trail that leads to a rock shelter and other geologic formations.

Note: Iron Ridge Campground will be closed for renovations during the 2012 camping season.

KEY INFORMATION

ADDRESS: 6518 State Route 93 Pedro, OH 45659

OPERATED BY: USDA Forest Service, Wayne National Forest, Ironton Ranger District

INFORMATION: (740) 534-6500; www.fs.usda.gov/wayne

RESERVATIONS: (877) 444-6777; recreation.gov

OPEN: April–October

SITES: Iron Ridge: 21 non-electric, 20 electric; Oak Hill: 8 non-electric, 32 electric

EACH SITE: Picnic table, fire ring, tent pad

ASSIGNMENT: Reservable sites; first come, first served

REGISTRATION: Self-registration station at bulletin board

FACILITIES: Showers, flush toilets, latrines, water spigots, swimming beach

PARKING: At each site

FEE: Iron Ridge and Oak Hill: $21 electric, $16 non-electric; senior and access pass $13 electric, $8 non-electric

ELEVATION: 600 feet

RESTRICTIONS: *Pets:* Must be leashed and attended
Fires: In fire ring
Alcohol: Prohibited
Vehicles: 2 per site
Other: Quiet hours 10 p.m.–6 a.m.; no nails or damage to trees; 8 persons per site

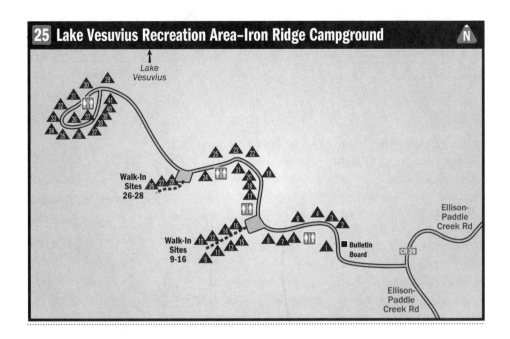

Lake
Vesuvius

30
29
31
32
41
40
33 37 39
36 38
34 35 36 37

25
23
22

Walk-In
Sites
26-28
26 27 28
24
21
20
18
17
19

6
4
3
2

Walk-In
Sites
9-16
10 12
14
16
15
8 7 5
1
11
13
9

Bulletin
Board
CR 29

Ellison-
Paddle
Creek Rd

Ellison-
Paddle
Creek Rd

GETTING THERE

From Ironton, travel north on OH 93 for 6.11 miles to CR 29 on the right. Follow CR 29 for 0.88 mile to a park road on the left. Follow this forest road to Oak Hill Campgrounds. Stay on CR 29 for another 1.28 miles to a road on the left to arrive at the Iron Ridge campground.

GPS COORDINATES

N38°36.282'
W82°37.931'

CAMPING ALONG the Ohio River is an exciting way to soak up some major river atmosphere. The campground at Leith Run is favored by a mix of camping enthusiasts, including tent campers, who have three sites dedicated to their method of camping. Paved roads cruise through the campground, where RVs like to tread but are not piled together like a mountain of aluminum-sided boxes. The 18 sites providing utilities rival a well-developed town, yet they're also spaced far enough from one another to welcome a family of tent campers to drop in between the rigs. Sites 11 and 19 sit on the well-mowed and maintained bank of the Ohio River, and because the focus is on the river, the occupants won't care what their neighbors are sleeping in. This place is as quiet, relaxed, and orderly as any campground that allows RVs.

Each site is equipped with a first-class fire ring/grill combo. There is something stirring about campfire smoke lingering along the banks of a grand river. Newer shower houses sit in the center of the open woodland campground and are well maintained—a welcome refresher after a day of catfishing or hiking the river and ridge trails. At the property's east side, a tent can be pitched on one of three sites that demand a 30-yard walk in. Site 21 on the Ohio River's edge is a popular site for tents. The river bank beckons campers to drag out a chair and sit a spell. If it wasn't for the occasional string of barges being pushed by with a tugboat, it would be easy to believe that at any moment a log raft with a straw-hat-wearing captain could come floating by.

Between the riverside sites of the campground's main section and site 21 sit a raised, wooden observation deck and a picnic shelter. This area is considered a day-use area, so expect to have a visitor or two pass by your tent site until darkness falls. Bring a pair of binoculars to this point and whittle away some time peering

> *Be mesmerized by the mighty but gentle Ohio River.*

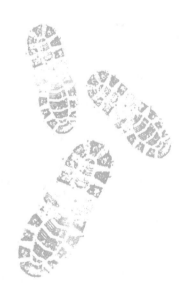

RATINGS

Beauty: ✩ ✩ ✩
Privacy: ✩ ✩ ✩
Spaciousness: ✩ ✩ ✩
Quiet: ✩ ✩ ✩
Security: ✩ ✩
Cleanliness: ✩ ✩ ✩ ✩

KEY INFORMATION

ADDRESS: 44400 State Route 7 New Matamoras, OH 45767

OPERATED BY: Marietta Unit, Athens Ranger Dist., U.S. Forest Service

INFORMATION: (740) 373-9055; www.fs.fed.us

RESERVATIONS: (877) 444-6777; recreation.gov

OPEN: May 27–October 10

SITES: 18 full service; 3 nonelectric tent sites

EACH SITE: Picnic table, fire ring, lantern posts

ASSIGNMENT: Reservable sites; first come, first served

REGISTRATION: Self-registration station at bulletin board

FACILITIES: Showers, flush toilets, playground, sports courts

PARKING: At each site, except campers at tent-only sites should park in lot next to shower house

FEE: $21 electric; $15 nonelectric; add $10 for reservation fee

ELEVATION: 615 feet

RESTRICTIONS: *Pets:* On leash only *Fires:* In fire ring *Alcohol:* Prohibited *Vehicles:* 2 per site, overflow parking available in lot *Other:* Quiet hours 10 p.m.–6 a.m.; downed wood may be gathered for firewood; 8 people maximum per site; 14-day stay limit

up and down the river. You will see critters visiting the riverbank to slurp a drink, and maybe even a close-up shot of a sternwheeler with waving tourists. Sites 20 and 22 are on the banks of the Ohio River tributary from which the recreation area gets its name—the Leith Run. A footpath leads from the heart of the campground to a fishing pier at the easternmost point of the property, where the tributary enters the river. Upstream from that confluence and the tent sites is an old boat launch ramp that is no longer in use, except by canoers and kayakers. Siltation has reduced the water depth here to not more than a couple feet.

Leith Run Recreation Area is a place to gain some needed rest and relaxation, but if hiking is your forte, consider tackling the 4-mile Scenic River Trail. The trail is accessible from the campground, crosses State Route 7 (marked with signage), and ends near the German Cemetery on County Road 9. The trail is well blazed with yellow and white diamonds as it winds up and around steep ridges with occasional vistas of the Ohio River. Rock outcroppings and sizable trees are trail highlights, and even if you trek up 1 mile before turning back, it will be worth the effort. Don't be surprised if a black bear scampers across the path in front of you, as this section of Wayne National Forest has several bear sightings each year.

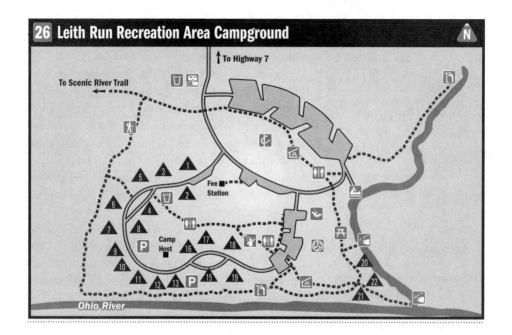

GETTING THERE

From I-77 Exit 1 in Marietta, travel east on OH 7 for 20.4 miles to the campground entrance on the right.

GPS COORDINATES

N39°26.986'
W81°8.784'

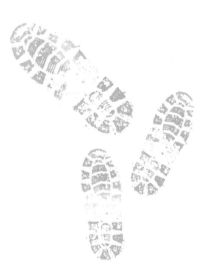

The sense of a remote Canadian lake atmosphere overcomes visitors here.

THE **MUSKINGUM WATERSHED** Conservancy District (MWCD) manages more than 8,000 square miles and 14 lakes throughout eastern Ohio. One of those lakes, Piedmont Lake and its surroundings, may be the most special of the group in regard to outdoor recreation with a dose of nostalgia. The MWCD was created to control flooding in the expansive watershed that feeds one river—the Muskingum River. The big job of planning and constructing dams began in the early 1930s. Although the dams were created for flood control and water conservation, they soon became playgrounds for outdoor adventurers. Piedmont became a favorite for many only a few years after its completion. Today, the atmosphere of a remote, relaxed wilderness location still exists and is appreciated. The campground is frequented by anglers and boaters. You'll see many pontoon boats moored at the marina or along the shoreline at the campground. The marina store is a neat place to see and feel the past. The interior décor gives the sense that you are at a remote Canadian lake lodge. The state record muskie hangs on the wall—a 55-pound trophy fish taken from the lake. The short drive down a fairly steep grade from OH 800 to the marina and campground seems like a time portal, with a lake paradise greeting those who make the travel back in time.

From the marina store, the campground is located just around the corner. There is only one road into the marina/campground area, which keeps traffic noise to a bare minimum. The campground rests in a cove, and when the wind comes out of the east, a cool lake breeze filters through the camp. Although the campground is inhabited by several seasonal campers, a fair share of overnight sites remain open for tenters. The lakeside sites are taken by seasonals, but a walkway for all campers passes between sites 6 and 7. A group of sites surrounded by the looping campground road, sites 47–56, are level and

RATINGS

Beauty: ✿ ✿
Privacy: ✿
Spaciousness: ✿ ✿
Quiet: ✿ ✿
Security: ✿ ✿ ✿
Cleanliness: ✿ ✿

provide the nearest access to the lake. At one end of this loop, near sites 47 and 56, is the primary shower house. Tent sites 79–89 offer the most solitude in this compact campground and are found on the northwest edge. This string of sites is spaced nicely along the base of a forested hill with an abundance of hardwood trees standing guard throughout all of the sites. Across the lane from these sites are sites 72–78, which are a touch shorter than sites 79–89 but are still separated from a row of full hook-up sites by a small, vegetation-covered stream. A drinking water spigot is situated across the lane from site 87 and near a playground. This campground in the cove is a pleasant place to rest your body after a day of boating around Piedmont Lake's 38 miles of gorgeous shoreline of rock and forest.

The campground and marina skirt the northwest stretch of the windy, coursing lake. Just north on OH 22, there is a well-maintained rest area and picnic facility. Hikers can also access the North Country Trail from that facility. The North Country Trail shares the same path with the Buckeye Trail at many points around Ohio, including this one. This portion of the established hiking trail leads from the rest area around the lower portion of three primary ridges that disappear into Piedmont Lake. The trail is maintained by volunteers of the Buckeye Trail Association. The view of the lake from the trail demands a camera. Be sure your camera battery is fully charged, as the 4.72-mile stretch of trail offers a multitude of photographic opportunities. At the 2.07-mile point from the rest area, a look at the lake's impressive length comes into view. If you go the full 4.72 miles of the Piedmont section, you will end up at Thin Lane, which connects to Marina Road. After 4.53 miles the trail passes near the most western edge of the campground. The trail is a quiet one, which works nicely with the Piedmont Lake time-warp theme.

KEY INFORMATION

ADDRESS: 32281 Marina Road Freeport, OH 43973

OPERATED BY: Muskingum Watershed Conservancy District

INFORMATION: (740) 922-3649 (this number reaches Tappan Lake Park, which manages Piedmont); www.mwcd.org/recreation

RESERVATIONS: First come, first served

OPEN: April–October

SITES: 86

EACH SITE: Picnic table, fire ring, electric

ASSIGNMENT: First come, first served

REGISTRATION: At Piedmont Marina store; if closed, self-registration at store

FACILITIES: Supply store, showers, flush toilets and latrine, drinking water; playground, direct access to the lake, boat rentals

PARKING: At each site

FEE: $26.50

ELEVATION: 920 feet

RESTRICTIONS: *Pets:* On leash only in designated areas *Fires:* In fire ring *Alcohol:* Not in public *Vehicles:* 1 per site *Other:* 2 tents per site; must be 18 to register for a site; quiet hours 11 p.m.–7 a.m.; dead wood may be gathered from ground for firewood

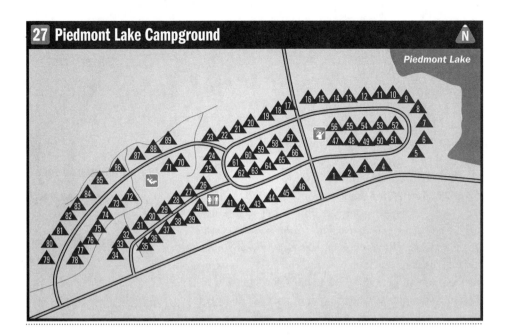

Piedmont Lake

GETTING THERE

From I-77 north, northeast of Cambridge, take Exit 47 to OH 22. Travel east 20.28 miles to OH 800, and then proceed south 0.59 mile to Marina Road (CR 893). Take Marina Road 1.04 miles to Piedmont Marina (also camp store).

GPS COORDINATES

N40°9.973'
W81°13.60'

28
SALT FORK
STATE PARK

SALT FORK STATE PARK is Ohio's largest state park. Not only does the park earn this title because of its expansive spread, but also because of the plethora of natural recreation and exploration options here. The park's name was derived from a salt source utilized by Native Americans. The region boasts several geographical highlights that attract visitors year-round today. The forested ravines are believed by some to be the home of the Ohio Grassman—Ohio's version of Bigfoot. The natural landscape here provides the perfect tent-camping environment.

This countryside welcomes those who enjoy a multi-mile hike among moist sandstone boulders decorating forest hills, as well as those who prefer a day on the water with rod and reel, or making wakes with a paddle or an outboard engine. An 18-hole golf course lies in the park's center, as does a mini-golf course at the beach. The variety of activities around the park is as diverse as the camping. A 200-plus-site modern campground provides amenity-rich camping, but for the tent camper, the park has just the place for a quiet night's sleep and a peaceful day of relaxation—an isolated, primitive campground, disconnected from the main campground.

Salt Fork's primitive campground was once a collection of small picnic areas. Because of its location off the main road and away from the park's major attractions, the ridge was transformed by park managers into five small groups of spacious, tent-only campsites. These sites require a small walk to the site from a paved parking area. The longest distance from parking to campsite is only 40 yards. Entering the primitive camping area, a picnic area sits on the left side of the paved road. Immediately on the right is Primitive Camp (PC) 5, which hosts three sites dispersed on a small rise iced with a few trees. Only three sites exist in PC5, but if camping with a few friends, your small group could have that section to yourselves.

> *Ohio's largest state park, yet quiet camping exists here.*

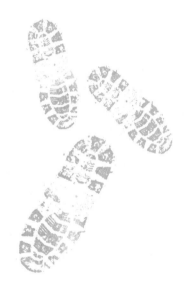

RATINGS

Beauty: ✩ ✩ ✩
Privacy: ✩ ✩ ✩
Spaciousness: ✩ ✩
Quiet: ✩ ✩ ✩ ✩
Security: ✩ ✩ ✩ ✩
Cleanliness: ✩ ✩ ✩

KEY INFORMATION

ADDRESS: 14755 Cadiz Road Lore City, OH 43755-9602

OPERATED BY: ODNR Division of Parks

INFORMATION: (740) 432-1508; www.dnr.state .oh.us/parks

RESERVATIONS: First come, first served

OPEN: Year-round; camp store closed Dec.– March; one heated shower building open in main campground

SITES: 24

EACH SITE: Fire ring, shared picnic tables

ASSIGNMENT: First come, first served

REGISTRATION: At main campground office

FACILITIES: Pit latrines, drinking water, dishwater disposal; all amenities at main campground available for campers at primitive sites (showers, flush toilets, laundry, beach, boat launch)

PARKING: At designated parking areas (short walk to sites)

FEE: $17

ELEVATION: 999 feet

RESTRICTIONS: *Pets:* On leash only *Fires:* In fire ring *Alcohol:* Prohibited *Vehicles:* 2 per site; no parking on grass or along road *Other:* Quiet hours 10 p.m.–7 a.m.; limit 6 persons per site; gathering firewood prohibited

Across the road and a dozen yards down the park road is PC4. This four-site section is tucked into the woods surrounding an open area that includes a pit latrine, drinking fountain, and dishwater disposal basin. Site 4 is the farthest from the road, and most private. The terrain slopes slightly under PC4 but is not a problem. With the closeness of trees and a few spreading shrubs here, a large tent should be avoided.

Back across the road and next to PC5 is PC3. The five sites here are spread out across the peak of a wide ridge that slopes away from the road. Sites 1 and 5 are hidden from the road, offering the most privacy. The road leading through the primitive campground is seldom traveled, so road noise is not an issue. The only other motor noise that may be heard comes from boats cruising the 3,000-acre Salt Fork Lake, at the bottom of the ridge on which the campground is perched. Because of the heavy forest cover, views of the lake from this campground only occur when the deciduous trees have shed their leaves for the season.

Six hundred feet down and across the road from PC3 is PC2. This section holds the most amenities of the primitive camp. The four sites of PC2 are situated in the four corners of the section, with pit latrines, a water fountain, and dishwater basin in the center. The water fountain is located next to site 1, the site nearest to the road. With eight-site PC1 across the road from PC2, PC2 receives the most foot traffic from campers using the restroom and obtaining drinking water. PC2's site 3 overlooks a wooded ravine. Various species of wildlife roam to the ridge top to meander around the campsites, so keep the camera handy and the snacks sealed away.

PC1 is at the end of the dead-end road. Eight sites in two rows roll away from the parking area. Site 4, at the end of the row on the right, distances itself from the rest by a few extra yards and rests at the ridgeline's perimeter. Although site 4 demands the longest walk from the car, the touch of solitude gained is worth it. At the end of PC1's parking area is the Gibson Farm trailhead, a 0.3-mile out–and-back path that passes by small caves and rock outcroppings.

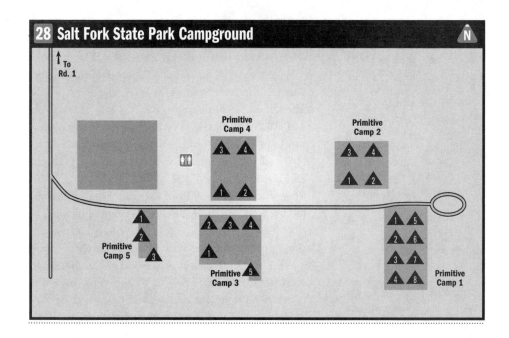

GETTING THERE

From I-77, Exit 47, north of Cambridge, follow OH 22 east 6.44 miles to park entrance on left. Travel Park Road 1 for 4.57 miles to Park Road 4 on the left. Follow Park Road 4 for 0.72 mile to left turn in the road. Bear left; campground signage will be on the right after passing a paved parking area on the left.

GPS COORDINATES

N40°7.526'
W81°30.420'

"One glance at Dow Lake and you'll want to pull over and soak up the atmosphere.

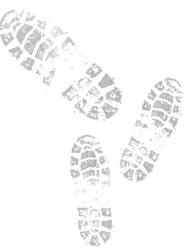

THE DRIVE TO STROUDS RUN STATE PARK includes a small jaunt through Athens, Ohio, with a few sharp turns and stops. For first-time visitors, the effort to find the little park may seem troublesome—until they arrive at the lake and then the campground. CR 20 follows the shoreline of the upper end of the 161-acre Dow Lake before leading to TR 212, which leads to the campground (signs posted). One glance at the lake and you'll want to pull over, throw down a picnic blanket, and soak up the lake atmosphere. This small lake is surrounded by hardwood forest, except for the northeast shoreline, which hosts a sandy beach and picnic area. During spring, summer, and fall, the lake is busy with small boats of anglers and paddling enthusiasts—many of them young people from the nearby Ohio University in Athens, the first college in the Northwest Territory. The campground is also frequented by the college kids, but they seem to respect campground regulations.

The campground lies in a valley with a small stream running at the base of the east hillside. Half of the sites sit sandwiched between the stream and campground road. The sites on the other side of the campground road have TR 212 to their backs. Normally a quiet road, TR 212 doesn't cause too much distraction from quiet camping. Shade falls on most of the campground sites, with sections of sunshine beaming through during midday. Sites 1 and 2 are in full sun, while sites 17–20 have ample space and plenty of shade. There is a drinking water–spigot at site 25. After reaching the cul-de-sac and heading back out, sites 40, 41, and 42 on the right sit near the Homestead Trail access; this trail blends into the Vista Point Trail. The Homestead Trail is tough at times, but the view overlooking Dow Lake is worth the trip—don't forget to bring a camera. The Vista Point Trail is accessed near the amphitheater on the left as you pull into the campground. A footbridge crosses Labath Run and

RATINGS

Beauty: ☆
Privacy: ☆ ☆
Spaciousness: ☆ ☆
Quiet: ☆ ☆
Security: ☆ ☆
Cleanliness: ☆ ☆

soon ascends to the overlook. Keep an eye out for the Indian mound 0.95 mile from the Vista Point trailhead.

A small store near the boat ramp on Dow Lake (0.24 mile from the campground entrance) handles boat rentals, as well as vending ice cream to refuel paddlers returning from a cruise on the lake. The fishing in Dow Lake varies in species and access. Most of the lake's edges are steep and inaccessible by foot, but the South Lakeview Trail does put the adventurous angler in position at several points, to make a few casts. The trailhead can be found by beginning where TR 212 turns off CR 20 and traveling west for 0.83 mile to the parking area on the left. Hikers and bikers share the 3-mile trail, but there are more of the first than the second. Rainbow trout are stocked in the lake each spring, and the locals work the lake pretty hard for the first week following the stocking. A few hundred of the trout go deep, however, and can occasionally be caught for a couple months afterward—healthy trout make a fine camp dinner.

Note: To register for a campsite, you must be 18 years old or provide a park officer with written consent from a parent or legal guardian.

KEY INFORMATION

ADDRESS: 11661 State Park Road
Athens, OH 45701

OPERATED BY: ODNR Division of Parks

INFORMATION: (740) 592-2302 (Reaches Burr Oak State Park, which handles Strouds Run State Park's calls); www.dnr .state.oh.us/parks

RESERVATIONS: (866) 644-6727; www.ohio.reserve world.com

OPEN: Year-round

SITES: 78 nonelectric

EACH SITE: Picnic table, fire ring

ASSIGNMENT: Reservable sites; walk-in sites first come, first served

REGISTRATION: At self-registration station at entrance

FACILITIES: Latrines, drinking water, dump station, playground, pay phone

PARKING: At each site

FEE: $17 April– October, $15 November–March; January–April no reservations taken; all sites are first come, first served

ELEVATION: 668 feet

RESTRICTIONS: *Pets:* On leash only
Fires: In fire ring
Alcohol: Prohibited
Vehicles: 1 per site
Other: Quiet hours 10 p.m.–7 a.m.; gathering firewood prohibited; must register before occupying site; no ATVs

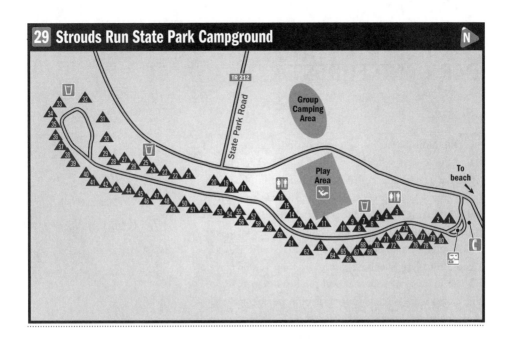

GETTING THERE

Traveling southeast on OH 33 north of Athens, take the OH 13/OH 550, Chauncey/Amesville exit. At the traffic light, turn right onto Columbus Road. Travel 1.82 miles to North Lancaster Road on the left. Go 0.16 mile and make a sharp left turn onto Columbia Avenue; travel 1.03 miles to CR 20 (Stroud's Run Road). Go 0.39 mile to the dead end, and then turn right and drive 3.1 miles to TR 212. Turn left and drive 0.08 mile to the campground entrance on the left.

GPS COORDINATES

N39°21.305'
W82°2.378'

TAR HOLLOW STATE PARK AND FOREST

THE **ABUNDANCE** of access possibilities to one of Ohio's best wilderness areas is why Tar Hollow State Park and State Forest is easily explored. Campers have access to the deep ravines and dense woodlands with 24 hiking miles, 21 backpacking miles, and 2.5 miles of mountain bike trails. Plus, 17 miles of paved roads and 14 miles of gravel roads offer scenic views of Ohio's third-largest state forest (more than 16,000 acres). The abundance of shortleaf and pitch pines growing on the ridges were once a source of pine tar for early settlers, the source of the park's name.

Spending one night in Tar Hollow's forests creates the desire for at least one more. The campground's deep woodland environment, along with the excellent trail and road access, makes the park a perfect multiday retreat. There is truly not a bad site in the six camping locations. Driving in on Tar Hollow Road from OH 327, the first campground option will be on the left in 1.17 miles. Nine sites encompass a stone parking area at the base of 15-acre Pine Lake's dam. The lake's spillway delivers a trickle of water regularly, but it picks up volume during rains. The released water doesn't impact the camping, as the water is contained in a 5-yard-wide ditch. The sites closest to the dam, sites 87, 88, and 95, fill first on the weekends. A moderate walk up the mowed grass–covered dam produces decent fishing. These sites are nonelectric, well spaced, and partially shaded.

Travel 0.45 mile farther on Tar Hollow Road to locate the beach (with one campsite between the beach and a picnic area), general store (camper registration and free Wi-Fi), miniature golf, and bike and boat rentals. This is the hub of activity and information for the campgrounds, especially for camping families staying in the two main campgrounds just ahead. Across the road from the beach entrance are two sites sitting back in a small, wooded

> *Ohio's third-largest state forest surrounds Tar Hollow State Park.*

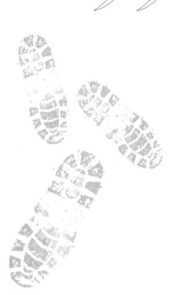

RATINGS

Beauty: ✿ ✿ ✿
Privacy: ✿ ✿ ✿
Spaciousness: ✿ ✿
Quiet: ✿ ✿ ✿
Security: ✿ ✿ ✿ ✿
Cleanliness: ✿ ✿ ✿

ADDRESS:	16396 Tar Hollow Rd., Laurelville, OH 43135
OPERATED BY:	ODNR Division of State Parks
INFORMATION:	(740) 887-4818; www.dnr.state.oh.us/parks
RESERVATIONS:	(866) 644-6727; www.ohio.reserve world.com
OPEN:	Year-round with limited amenities
SITES:	12 walk-in; 5 backpack; 11 nonelectric; 71 electric
EACH SITE:	Picnic table, fire ring
ASSIGNMENT:	Reservable sites; walk-in sites first come, first served
REGISTRATION:	At store (log cabin); self-registration info outside
FACILITIES:	Showers, flush toilets, laundry, store, boat ramp, swimming beach, bike and boat rental, game room, minigolf, nature center
PARKING:	At each site, but parking area for walk-in sites
FEE:	$22 nonelectric and walk-in; $25 electric; deduct $1 from fee Sun.–Thurs.; $2 off in winter
ELEVATION:	814 feet
RESTRICTIONS:	*Pets:* On leash only *Fires:* In fire ring *Alcohol:* Prohibited *Vehicles:* 1 per site *Other:* Quiet hours 10 p.m.–8 a.m.; gathering firewood prohibited; limit 6 persons per site

cove—rightly named the General Cove sites. The next right off Tar Hollow Road leads to Logan Hollow Campground. The 41 electric sites, the most rustic of the 71 electric sites of Tar Hollow State Park, are stretched out along the narrow valley, with steep ridges rising up on both sides. The sites on the left going in (sites 38–50) sit along a stream that keeps cool, thanks to the heavy tree canopy overhead. A short spur road off the Logan Hollow road holds sites 67–71. These five sites offer a quiet option if the main sections get busy. In the next hollow over from Logan Hollow is Ross Hollow Campground. All 28 electric sites have paved parking pads and are normally taken by RVs. A heated shower house and pay phone sit at the entrance to this section.

Back on Tar Hollow Road, travel 1.19 miles up a windy, narrow section of the road also called Park Road 10. You will arrive at the top of a ridge (330 feet higher in elevation) that overlooks the main campgrounds. Perched on that ridgetop is North Ridge Walk In Campground. The drive up the mountain to this remote campground may give the impression the road leads to nowhere, but the destination is one any tent camper will appreciate. Twelve sites circle a 1-acre clearing on the peak of the forested ridge. The sites could be enhanced with a few more yards between them, but because this campground is so out of the way, it goes somewhat unnoticed—that's a good thing.

The first site is only a few yards from the gravel parking area and bulletin board. Sites 101–106 are the cream of the crop, with autumn and spring views of distant ridges that are filled with dew clouds in the mornings. The other six sites are strung along the lower side of the clearing but are still worthy because of the sense of serenity felt there.

For an even more deep-forest-camping experience, follow the park road out to South Ridge Road (Park Road 3), take a left, and drive south 1.47 miles to the fire tower. East of the fire tower parking area are five backpacking sites just out of sight on the opposite side of a small latrine. Camping here costs $5 per adult. The North Country Trail passes through the park at this point using Tar Hollow's Logan Trail. If you put your boots to any of Tar Hollow's trails, keep an eye out for

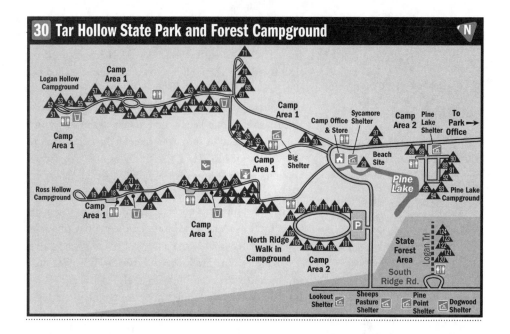

timber rattlesnakes. The rattlers are at home on the dry, rocky ridgetops of the park. Timber rattlers are found in only seven counties in Ohio, and Tar Hollow lies in three of those counties.

GETTING THERE

From Adelphi, travel 7.36 miles south on OH 327 to the park entrance on the right.

GPS COORDINATES

N39°23.018'
W82°44.777'

31
WOLF RUN
STATE PARK

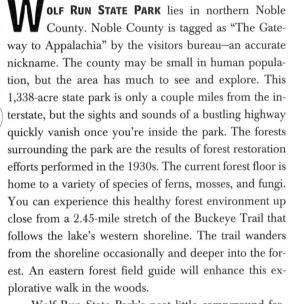

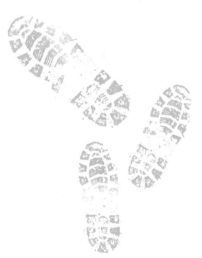

> *This quiet, beautiful park is easily accessible from the interstate.*

WOLF RUN STATE PARK lies in northern Noble County. Noble County is tagged as "The Gateway to Appalachia" by the visitors bureau—an accurate nickname. The county may be small in human population, but the area has much to see and explore. This 1,338-acre state park is only a couple miles from the interstate, but the sights and sounds of a bustling highway quickly vanish once you're inside the park. The forests surrounding the park are the results of forest restoration efforts performed in the 1930s. The current forest floor is home to a variety of species of ferns, mosses, and fungi. You can experience this healthy forest environment up close from a 2.45-mile stretch of the Buckeye Trail that follows the lake's western shoreline. The trail wanders from the shoreline occasionally and deeper into the forest. An eastern forest field guide will enhance this explorative walk in the woods.

Wolf Run State Park's neat little campground features three sections sitting like a crown atop five adjoining finger ridges. After a quick stop at the camp store/registration center, you will likely see RVers at the sites straight ahead. Turn right at the intersection and follow the main campground road past two sections of sites on the left, and then follow the road around and down a long hill to the best tent sites at Wolf Run. At the bottom of the hill and the lake's edge are sites 22–26, titled as premium lakeside sites—and they are. These five sites have panoramic views of the picturesque lake, and a few steps from the site take you to the water's edge. The sites are roomy enough for a large tent, but with such a pretty lake environment, little time will be spent in the tent. The lake has a 10-hp limit, so you can paddle it without the concern of overcoming 3-foot wakes. While sitting at your site at dusk and dawn, you may spot a Great Blue Heron wading in the shallows in search of food. Rainbow trout are released into the lake each March, which

RATINGS

Beauty: ✩ ✩ ✩
Privacy: ✩ ✩
Spaciousness: ✩ ✩
Quiet: ✩ ✩
Security: ✩ ✩ ✩
Cleanliness: ✩ ✩ ✩

draws a decent number of anglers. From this group of sites, a 1.1-mile hiking trail leads to the beach east of the campground.

Traveling back up the hill on the main campground road, you'll find sites 27–36 on the right and situated along the rim of a lake cove. These sites are sloping but manageable for tent camping. A steep walk from each site through the forested banks will lead to the lake. Across the road from site 30 are a drinking water spigot and latrine. Once on top of the hill, take the branch to the right between sites 44 and 67. Go to the cul-de-sac to find sites 51–56. These sites are a bit tight but can accommodate a four-person tent. During green leaf season, the lake is hidden by vegetation, but in the early spring and fall, campers will enjoy a view of the lake and cool breezes. A latrine is near site 56, and a shower house sits between sites 46 and 45, which you passed on the right after turning onto the branch road. This shower house is the closer of the two in the campground to the sites highlighted so far.

Return to the main campground road and go straight to a cul-de-sac surrounded by sites 126–133. You will pass a group of sites on the right getting to that point, but those are usually filled with RVs. Sites 126–133 have an overlook of the lake and dam. The sites are not so spacious, but the view is worth the effort to squeeze your tent onto the site. These sites are mostly sunny, but westerly winds keep them fresh.

For a peek at some history that has affected everyone's lives, jump back on I-77 and go south to Exit 25. Drive 1.8 miles east on OH 78 to the junction of OH 564. There you will find the first oil well in North America. It's a historical site that is protected by a fence, but you can view it. The well, created in 1814, is still lined with a hollow sycamore log that is visible sticking up above the well today. An on-site historical marker tells the rest of the story.

KEY INFORMATION

ADDRESS:	16170 Wolf Run Rd. Caldwell, OH 43724-9503
OPERATED BY:	ODNR Division of Parks
INFORMATION:	(740) 732-5035; www.dnr.state.oh.us/parks
RESERVATIONS:	(866) 644-6727; www.ohio.reserveworld.com
OPEN:	Year-round; non-electric sites closed Dec. 8–Apr. 1
SITES:	71 electric; 67 nonelectric
EACH SITE:	Picnic table, fire ring
ASSIGNMENT:	Reservable sites; walk-in sites first come, first served
REGISTRATION:	At camp store; self-registration station on front of store
FACILITIES:	Store, showers, flush toilets and latrines, laundry, playground, sports courts, boat ramp, nature center
PARKING:	At each site
FEE:	$23 electric; $19 nonelectric; $20 nonelectric premium site (lakeside); $2 off in winter; $1 off Sun.–Thurs.
ELEVATION:	890 feet
RESTRICTIONS:	*Pets:* At sites 44–50 and 57–103 only and on leash *Fires:* In fire ring *Alcohol:* Prohibited *Vehicles:* 2 per site *Other:* Quiet hours 10 p.m.–8 a.m.; gathering firewood prohibited; 14-day stay limit

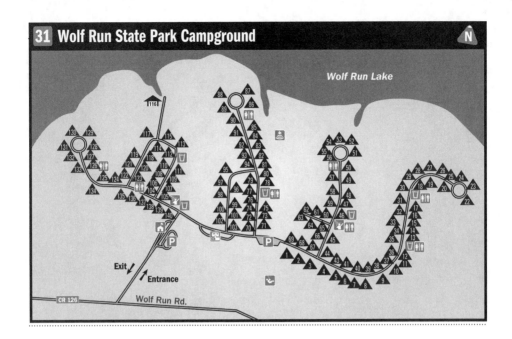

GETTING THERE

From I-77 Exit 28 in Belle Valley, go south on OH 821 for 0.44 mile to OH 215 on the left. Travel 0.97 mile to CR 126 on the left and go 0.33 mile to the park entrance on the right.

GPS COORDINATES

N39°47.3742'
W81°32.4297'

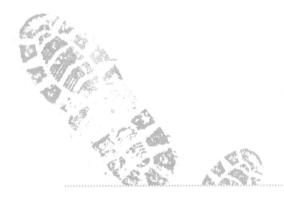
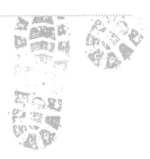

SOUTHWEST

32 GERMANTOWN METROPARK

ONLY **20** MINUTES from Dayton is a chunk of wilderness consisting of deep, scenic ravines that contain the Twin Creek, a tributary to the Great Miami River. A dam on Twin Creek controls any flooding and offers a great view of the park. Fossil hunting is permitted below the dam, where a canoe launch site is located—just follow the signage. The 1,655-acre Germantown Metropark is well known to children of the region, whose schools make frequent fieldtrips here. It's always refreshing to see kids knee-deep in nature. Sixteen miles of hiking trails weave through the park, while a paved park road courses through an old forest and a clean creek—both sustaining wildlife year-round. The park road is on the west side of Conservancy Road, just north of the dam, and has several pullover areas that lead to a fishing pond and a scenic overlook.

Spending a night immersed in the park's beautiful landscape is icing on the camper's adventure cake. There are two options for car camping here, and both offer a rare method of doing so, as there are no individual sites but one open site with a 6-foot-wide, steel fire ring in the center. On the park's eastern side is the Old Mill Campsite, not far from the Germantown Dam. A small, paved parking area that can handle only four vehicles sits next to Old Mill Road and features a small firewood supply shed, with free firewood for campers' use. Across the road from the parking area is a signpost marking the crossing of the Twin Valley Trail (TVT). The TVT is a backpacking trail that connects with the Germantown Metropark and the Twin Creek Metropark, which is south of Germantown.

Down a slight slope from the parking area is the shared camping area, measuring approximately 75 feet by 100 feet. A set of wood steps leading to a pit latrine are located on the grassy campsite's north side. The campsite is surrounded by forest, and there's a creek on

> *Spend a night immersed in this park's beautiful landscape.*

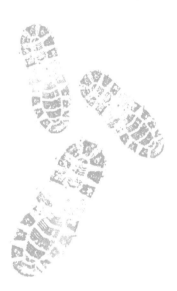

RATINGS

Beauty: ✩ ✩ ✩
Privacy: ✩ ✩ ✩ ✩
Spaciousness: ✩ ✩ ✩ ✩
Quiet: ✩ ✩ ✩ ✩
Security: ✩ ✩ ✩
Cleanliness: ✩ ✩ ✩

ADDRESS: 7173 Old Mill Road Germantown, OH 45327

OPERATED BY: Five Rivers Metroparks, Dayton

INFORMATION: (937) 275-7275; www.metroparks .org

RESERVATIONS: (937) 277-4374, Monday–Friday, 9 a.m.–4 p.m.; outdoors@ metroparks.org; must be made at least 1 week in advance

OPEN: Year-round

SITES: 1 large shared site

EACH SITE: Picnic table, center fire ring

ASSIGNMENT: By reservation only

REGISTRATION: Self-registration; display provided permit

FACILITIES: Pit latrine, fire-wood supply shelter

PARKING: Parking area at campground

FEE: Free

ELEVATION: 759 feet at Old Mill Campsite; 913 feet at Shimps Hollow Group Camp

RESTRICTIONS: *Pets:* On leash only
Fires: In fire ring
Alcohol: Prohibited
Vehicles: At parking area
Other: No firewood brought in, fire-wood provided; no amplified music

the far eastern side. The large fire ring near the campsite's center invites campers to sit a spell on the two log benches nearby. Two picnic tables are also set about the big site. A few trees spread about the site break it up when multiple camps are needed. The campsites don't get a lot of company, so you may just have the whole site to yourself. At the dead end of Old Mill Road is a picnic area that attracts day users. A trail leads from the picnic area for a circle hike through the Bob Siebenthaler Natural Area—a well-maintained woodland.

The second site is the Shimps Hollow Group Camp, across the metropark in the southwest corner of the property, off Boomershine Road. A gravel lane runs about a quarter mile from the road to the campsite parking area. This site also has one large fire ring, five picnic tables, and a latrine near the parking area. The site itself is approximately 75 feet by 400 feet and sprawls out under mature trees. Although the site is titled a group camp, individual campers are permitted to use the site if it's not fully reserved. The site sits at the edge and center of two hollows, hence its name. Both wooded hollows lead deep into the park toward the Orange Trail. The Orange Trail is a 6.8-mile hiking trail—if you only have time to take one of the park's seven trails, this is the one.

The park's fantastic nature center, north of the campsite on Boomershine Road, is worth a visit. (Water for camping is available here). From here, head north on the Orange Trail, which drops over the edge of the creek valley. The trail will pass the park's northern boundary before turning south on the valley's east side. The hardwood forest rimming the valley warrants frequent stops, so plan to spend a full day doing the trail. The trail turns west at the dam before turning back north again. Before you make it back to the nature center, you will have walked among one of the oldest forests surviving in the state today. Take many photos of this old-growth forest, for you may not see such a display of nature in Ohio again.

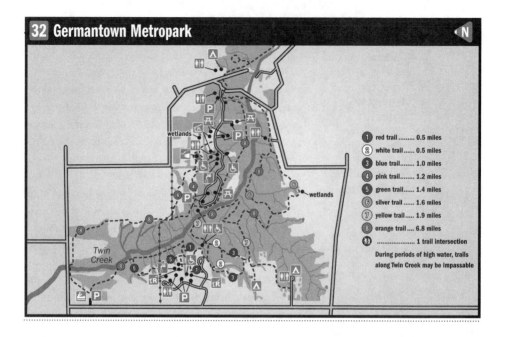

wetlands

wetlands

Twin
Creek

1	red trail .... 0.5 miles
2	white trail ...... 0.5 miles
3	blue trail .... 1.0 miles
4	pink trail .... 1.2 miles
5	green trail ...... 1.4 miles
6	silver trail ...... 1.6 miles
7	yellow trail ..... 1.9 miles
8	orange trail .... 6.8 miles
🚶	.... 1 trail intersection

During periods of high water, trails
along Twin Creek may be impassable

GETTING THERE

From Germantown, follow
OH 725 west for 2.21 miles
to Conservancy Road on the
right. Travel 1.59 miles north
to Old Mill Road on the
right. Follow Old Mill Road
0.15 mile to the Old Mill
Campsite on the left.

GPS COORDINATES

OLD MILL CAMPSITE:
N39°38.360'
W84°23.991'

SHIMPS HOLLOW GROUP CAMP:
N39°37.962'
W84°25.857'

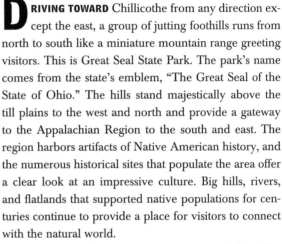

33
GREAT SEAL
STATE PARK

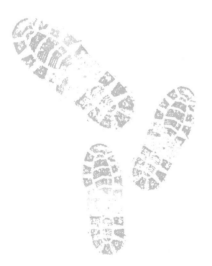

> *A range of majestic hills contains hundreds of years of Native American history.*

DRIVING TOWARD Chillicothe from any direction except the east, a group of jutting foothills runs from north to south like a miniature mountain range greeting visitors. This is Great Seal State Park. The park's name comes from the state's emblem, "The Great Seal of the State of Ohio." The hills stand majestically above the till plains to the west and north and provide a gateway to the Appalachian Region to the south and east. The region harbors artifacts of Native American history, and the numerous historical sites that populate the area offer a clear look at an impressive culture. Big hills, rivers, and flatlands that supported native populations for centuries continue to provide a place for visitors to connect with the natural world.

Halfway up Sugarloaf Mountain, rounded up like circled wagons, sit this park's small campground, with 15 sites. A shelter house and picnic area are located inside the campground loop. The shelter house is near the campground entrance, so picnickers aren't a bother to campers. Sites 1–10 are spread widely around the entire campground road loop. The campground covers approximately four acres of closely mowed lawn with a few trees here and there, and the outer sites are placed against outer edges of the clearing. Sites 11–15 are on the inside of the loop, starting near the picnic shelter. These five sites receive full sun all day.

As the loop makes the turn at the top of the slope, sites 6 and 7 sit hidden a few shady yards from three oak trees and the trees surrounding the open meadow. Each site has a gravel parking pad that can easily accommodate two vehicles. The sites were built to accommodate a horse trailer and tow vehicle, as this campground also serves as an equestrian camp (although riders are restricted to the 10 outskirt sites). A picket line for tethering horses runs along the back side of sites 1–10. The park managers enforce strict rules for owners to clean up after their animals.

RATINGS

Beauty: ✩ ✩ ✩
Privacy: ✩ ✩
Spaciousness: ✩ ✩ ✩
Quiet: ✩ ✩
Security: ✩ ✩
Cleanliness: ✩ ✩ ✩

A latrine and water spigot are only a few yards from the self-registration station, as is a wooden trailhead sign, signaling the three trails accessible from that one point: Sugarloaf Mountain, with yellow blazes and 2.1 miles long; the Shawnee Ridge, with blue blazes and 7.8 miles long; and the Mount Ives, with red blazes and 6.4 miles long. All of the trails traversing the jutting hills of Great Seal State Park are categorized as strenuous. The Sugarloaf Mountain trail rises to the mountain's peak, leading hikers on a 500-foot ascent in less than a quarter mile. A trail map is a necessity. Trail trekking is the main adventure here, and several of the trails are multiuse, supporting hikers, equestrians, and mountain bikers.

At the eastern base of Sugarloaf Mountain is the site of the outdoor historical drama *Tecumseh!*, performed June–early September at the Sugarloaf Mountain Amphitheater. For more Native American history, a visit to the Mound City/Hopewell Cultural Group National Historic Park will provide hours of learning. The park is located 1 mile north of Chillicothe on OH 104. Walk among 23 burial mounds and view artifacts discovered on the protected property displayed in the museum. A stroll along the Scioto River, which flows along the park's eastern boundary, demands a few moments' pause to let the mind consider how life was here a few hundred years ago.

ADDRESS: 4908 Marietta Road Chillicothe, OH 45601

OPERATED BY: ODNR Division of State Parks

INFORMATION: (740) 887-4818 (Tar Hollow State Park handles this park's calls); www.dnr .state.oh.us/parks

RESERVATIONS: (866) 644-6727; www.ohio.reserve world.com; if on site, call park office at (740) 887-4818 for same-day registration and use credit card, Monday–Friday

OPEN: Closed January– February

SITES: 15 nonelectric

EACH SITE: Picnic table, fire ring

ASSIGNMENT: Reservable sites

REGISTRATION: Self-registration station at campground entrance

FACILITIES: Latrine, water supply, playground

PARKING: At each site

FEE: $19; $1 off Sunday–Thursday; $2 off in winter

ELEVATION: 867 feet

RESTRICTIONS: *Pets:* On leash only *Fires:* In fire ring *Alcohol:* Prohibited *Vehicles:* 2 per site *Other:* Quiet hours 10 p.m.–8 a.m.; gathering firewood prohibited; limit 6 persons per site

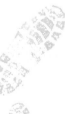

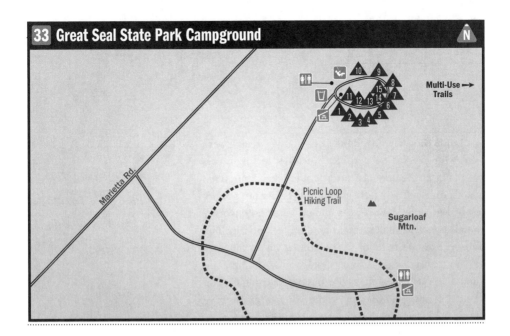

Multi-Use → Trails

Marietta Rd.

Picnic Loop
Hiking Trail

Sugarloaf
Mtn.

GETTING THERE

From Chillicothe, follow OH 159 north for 4.2 miles to Delano Road. Turn right and travel 0.97 mile to Marietta Road on the right. Travel south for 0.77 mile to park entrance on the left. Follow signage to the campground.

GPS COORDINATES

N39°24.139'
W82°56.474'

34
JOHN BRYAN
STATE PARK

Clifton

JOHN BRYAN STATE PARK is not only a scenic park with several geographical features for sightseers to enjoy, but the park also attracts avid hikers, mountain bikers, and cliff clingers. Hiking trails skirt the gorges, cut by the Little Miami River, and provide photo-worthy views, as well as challenging rock climbing and repelling for the extreme outdoor adventurer. With so much to do in and around the Clifton Gorge, a base camp is required, to catch a few needed winks before rising to head down the next trail. Before heading home, take a drive through or stroll in nearby Yellow Springs—a unique little town featuring artwork in its many galleries.

The campground lacks some common facilities such as showers, but its simplicity is appreciated. The entrance to the campground passes through a split-rail fence and the property opens out and up. The campground covers a rolling hill like a blanket. Halfway to the top of the hill on the right are sites 30–35. Those five sites have gravel parking pads attached to the paved lane, but the sites are 15 yards downhill from the parking pad. The slope is mostly open except for a few deciduous trees providing a hint of shade. These sites staked out on the grassy grade are nearly as wide as they are long, with lots of space for a big tent with comfy cots.

On the opposite side of the lane are sites 17–22, sitting near the top of the ridge, out in the open. As the long, looping lane turns, sites 27–29 sit on the edge of a thick forest. Sites 1–3 are next in line before the loop finishes the turn. Site 1 is inviting with space and the smell of oaks, but State Route 370 sneaks by in those woods, only a dozen yards away. Sites 4–11 are the kings of the hill, with paved parking pads and a wide view of the campground. RVers migrate to those sites, which keeps them primarily in one spot. The average camper at John Bryan State Park is in a tent, enjoying more than one day exploring the gorge.

> *The gorge here was cut by the Little Miami River, a State and National Scenic River.*

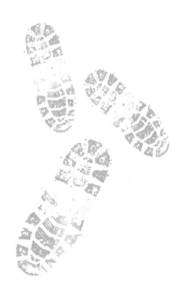

RATINGS

Beauty: ☆☆☆
Privacy: ☆☆☆
Spaciousness: ☆☆☆
Quiet: ☆☆☆
Security: ☆☆☆
Cleanliness: ☆☆☆

ADDRESS: 3790 State Route 370 Yellow Springs, OH 45387-9743

OPERATED BY: ODNR Division of State Parks

INFORMATION: (937) 767-1274; www.dnr.state .oh.us/parks

RESERVATIONS: (866) 644-6727; www.ohio.reserve world.com

OPEN: Year-round; limited facilities winter months; camp store closed November– mid-May

SITES: 50 nonelectric; 10 electric

EACH SITE: Picnic table, fire ring

ASSIGNMENT: Reservable sites; walk-in sites first come, first served

REGISTRATION: Self-registration station at camp- ground office, if office closed

FACILITIES: Pit latrines, camp store, pay phone, sports courts, play- ground

PARKING: At each site

FEE: $23 electric; $19 nonelectric

ELEVATION: 999 feet

RESTRICTIONS: *Pets:* On leash only
Fires: In fire ring
Alcohol: Prohibited
Vehicles: 2 per site
Other: Quiet hours 10 p.m.–8 a.m.; gathering firewood prohibited; limit 6 persons per site

The lane that ushers you into the campground cuts through its heart and, after cresting the hill, snakes to the left and right into the forest, skirting the campground's west side. Before the road enters the deeper forest, sites 58–60 sit on the left. Site 60 rests against the woods; from that point, a camper cannot see the majority of the campground and the campground can't see it. The lane passing by here is used by park personnel coming and going from a maintenance building in the woods past site 60. A water pump is available near the building. Sites 52–57 are east of site 60 and accessed from another looping lane opposite the first, larger one. Sites 55 and 56 offer the most space, with an open lawn area. At the middle of this loop is a smaller, connecting loop with sites 36–45. Sites 44 and 45 are on the outside of the little loop and near the edge of a steep ravine that carries the Little Miami River, 150 feet below. On breezy days, these sites catch a refreshing draft filtering up from the valley. A trail leads away from near site 38 and descends the ravine before arriving at the parking area of the lower picnic area. From there, a network of trails follows the river gorge for 2 miles.

From the campground entrance, take a right and then a left; bypass the day-use lodge on the left, pull over, and park at the Wingo Picnic Area. Lace up your hiking boots and hit the trail that leaves the south side of the picnic area and soon joins the North Rim trail. This will put you in the middle of the rock climbing and repelling area—to either rope up or simply observe.

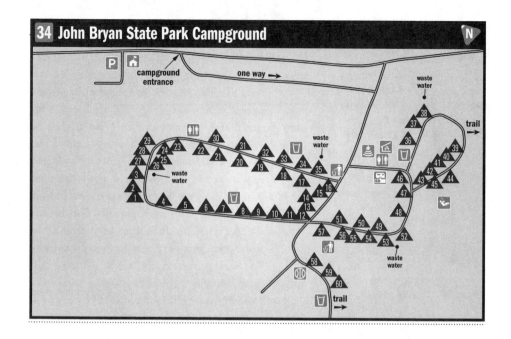

GETTING THERE

From Springfield, from I-70 Exit 52, follow US 68 south for 6.62 miles to OH 343 and turn left at the traffic light. Go east 0.96 mile to OH 370 (Bryan Park Road) and turn right. Travel south 1.1 miles to the park entrance and turn left. The campground office and sites are 500 feet ahead.

GPS COORDINATES

N39°47.348'
W83°51.955'

35
MIAMI WHITEWATER FOREST

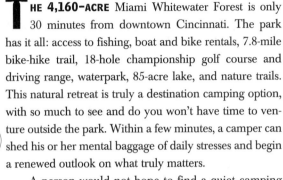

> *A recreational retreat 30 minutes from Cincinnati but without the metro mayhem.*

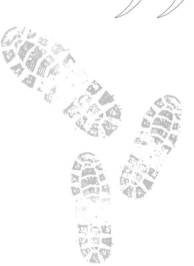

THE 4,160-ACRE Miami Whitewater Forest is only 30 minutes from downtown Cincinnati. The park has it all: access to fishing, boat and bike rentals, 7.8-mile bike-hike trail, 18-hole championship golf course and driving range, waterpark, 85-acre lake, and nature trails. This natural retreat is truly a destination camping option, with so much to see and do you won't have time to venture outside the park. Within a few minutes, a camper can shed his or her mental baggage of daily stresses and begin a renewed outlook on what truly matters.

A person would not hope to find a quiet camping spot within a few miles of a metropolitan area, or in a busy, county park—but it exists at Miami Whitewater Forest. A cone-shaped hill rises 100 feet to the west of the lake, which shares the park's name. The hill supports 46 campsites from the top to the bottom. Even during the peak of park visitation, midsummer, the campground remains a quiet retreat with some vacancy. The paved, one-way, campground loop lane heads uphill at the campground entrance. Sites flank both sides of the road that runs nearly one-half mile through the forested hill.

Sites 101–110 sit on the upslope, on individual shelves of gravel parking pads and small open areas that can accommodate a medium-sized tent at best. As the campground lane nears the peak, site 113 on the right is the last site on that side, until the lane winds around and descends 40 yards to the lower level and the remaining sites. Across the lane from site 113 are sites 114 and 115. These three sites offer views to the east and west when the trees have shed their leaves for the year. A steady breeze refreshes these higher sites, which are often unoccupied, making this uphill stretch of sites the most laid-back.

The entire hill is covered with a young, deciduous forest, which receives songbirds' constant echoing songs.

RATINGS

Beauty: ✰ ✰ ✰
Privacy: ✰ ✰ ✰
Spaciousness: ✰ ✰
Quiet: ✰ ✰ ✰
Security: ✰ ✰ ✰ ✰
Cleanliness: ✰ ✰ ✰

Birders will develop sore neck muscles from following the birds as they dart from tree to tree. Site 116 is the first site on the right after arriving at the campground's lower level. Site 116 requires a 10-yard walk from the parking pad to the site; the pad provides some privacy from the next site and the lane. From that point on, around to the last site and behind, the sites on the outer right side of the looping lane are backed by a safety fence. The fence keeps campers from falling over a cliff and into the Dry Fork Whitewater River. To access the river, use the two picnic areas along Timberlakes Drive. The curve in the river at the picnic area below the campground has two long, narrow holes that hold catfish during the warm months.

Site 128 is shortened in depth because of the nearness of the fence to the site. Sites 138–144 become a little close, so expect to trade camping stories or the day's adventures with your neighbors. The last two sites, sites 145 and 146 (one on each side of the lane), open up with a bit more space and no neighbors on the exit side. Back at the campground entrance is a newly renovated shower house with flush toilets, a potable water spigot, and a bulletin board.

Turn right out of the campground, return to Timberlakes Drive, and go left. Along the road you will see paved pullovers, but stop at the Timberlakes Program Shelter on the left, near the top of the ridge. From there, find access to a nature trail with interpretative stations. The park district maintains an extensive nature conservation program. When registering for your campsite at the boathouse, step into the visitor center and grab a trail map.

KEY INFORMATION

ADDRESS:	9001 Mt. Hope Rd. Harrison, OH 45030
OPERATED BY:	Hamilton County Park District
INFORMATION:	(513) 367-9632; www.greatparks.org
RESERVATIONS:	(513) 851-2267; www.greatparks.org
OPEN:	March–October
SITES:	46 electric
EACH SITE:	Picnic table, fire ring
ASSIGNMENT:	Reservable; first come, first served
REGISTRATION:	At the boathouse located near the wet playground at the lake
FACILITIES:	Showers, flush toilets, nature center at visitor center, boat rentals, disc golf, 18-hole golf course, playground, wet playground
PARKING:	At each site
FEE:	$25 plus $3-per-day park-use fee
ELEVATION:	609 feet
RESTRICTIONS:	*Pets:* Maximum 2 per site *Fires:* In fire ring *Alcohol:* Prohibited *Vehicles:* 2 per site *Other:* Quiet hours 10 p.m.–9 a.m.; no cutting trees for firewood; at least one member of camping party must be 18 years old

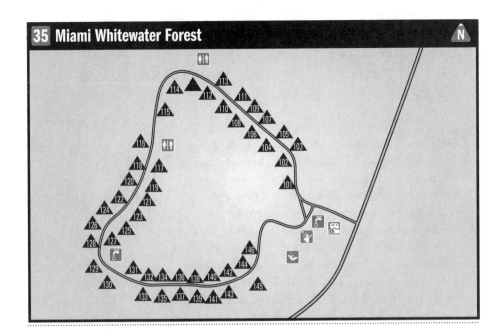

GETTING THERE

From Cincinnati's west side, take I-74 to Exit 3. Travel north 0.88 mile on Dry Fork Road to West Road and turn right. Follow West Road for 0.26 mile and turn left onto Timberlakes Drive. Travel 0.75 mile to Harbor Ridge Drive on the left. The campground entrance is ahead on the left.

GPS COORDINATES

N39°15.383'
W84°44.873'

PAINT CREEK STATE PARK

THE **PAINT CREEK REGION** lies at the edge of the Appalachian Plateau, marking the boundary between Ohio's hilly eastern section and the flatter western segment. The 1,200-acre Paint Creek Lake is a huge attraction at Paint Creek State Park, but surrounding the park there's still much to explore. The Seip Mound State Memorial lies 2.84 miles east of Bainbridge. The mound, more than 30 feet tall and 240 feet long, was built by Hopewell Indians starting around 100 B.C. Descriptive signage on site details the ways of the ancient people that once thrived throughout this region. South of the park on Cave Road, 1.36 miles from US 50, are the Highlands Nature Sanctuary and the Appalachian Forest Museum (**www.arcofappalachia.org**). For a $6 ticket, you will have access to 14 miles of hiking trails through a rocky gorge and forests with rare trees and plants—like walking through Ohio's wilds, centuries ago.

Sitting atop a split peninsula extending from Paint Creek Lake's eastern shore is a modern and very clean campground. Park friends are active year-round at the park, and it shows, with its paved pads and manicured lawns. This quiet campground hosts tent campers and RVs alike. A fully stocked camp store is the first stop at the campground's entrance. With a wide variety of outdoor pursuits to partake in here, it's worth a few moments to visit with the store's employees to get the scoop on current park events. Next to the camp store is a nature center that even big kids will enjoy.

Camping Area One is on the right past the store and spreads out on the peninsula's northern split. Sites 1–25 are popular with RVs. At the tip of Area One are several sites enhanced with wooden decks that overlook the lake. There are no designated trails leading from this point in the campground down to the lake. It's a steep drop from the campsites to the water, so ignore the urge to create a shortcut. Of the six sites with decks in Area

> *This park lies at the edge of Ohio's Appalachian Plateau.*

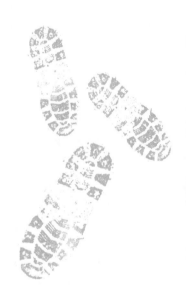

RATINGS

Beauty: ☆ ☆ ☆
Privacy: ☆ ☆
Spaciousness: ☆ ☆ ☆
Quiet: ☆ ☆
Security: ☆ ☆ ☆ ☆
Cleanliness: ☆ ☆ ☆ ☆

ADDRESS:	280 Taylor Road Bainbridge, OH 45612
OPERATED BY:	ODNR Division of State Parks
INFORMATION:	(937) 981-7061; www.dnr.state .oh.us/parks
RESERVATIONS:	(866) 644-6727; www.ohio.reserve world.com
OPEN:	Year-round; limited facilities in winter; camp store closed Nov.–March
SITES:	183 electric; primitive equestrian camp
EACH SITE:	Picnic table, fire ring
ASSIGNMENT:	Reservable sites; walk-in sites first come, first served
REGISTRATION:	Self-registration station at camp-ground office, if office closed
FACILITIES:	Showers, flush toi-lets, laundry, store, game room, boat launch, disc golf, miniature golf, swimming beach
PARKING:	At each site
FEE:	$25; $2 off winter; $1 off Sun.–Thurs.
ELEVATION:	910 feet
RESTRICTIONS:	*Pets:* On leash only; 2-pet maximum *Fires:* In fire ring *Alcohol:* Prohibited *Vehicles:* 2 per site; overflow parking near camp store *Other:* Quiet hours 10 p.m.–8 a.m.; gathering firewood prohibited; limit 6 persons per site

One, sites 37 and 38 are the only two that have ample space for pitching a tent. Following the area lane back to the main campground lane, site 57 on the right slopes a few yards downhill and sits off by itself a little. Site 62 on the left, opposite a rental cabin, escapes the lawn-like camping theme that describes most of the central sites and jumps into a small woodlot. A walk past three sites west from site 62 brings you to a shower house and drinking water.

The main campground lane leading from Area One to Area Two and Three has three sites on the right. Sites 67 and 69 offer quiet at the bottom of a short slope, even sitting within 70 yards of the camp store. Swing right into Area Three and onto the longest section of the peninsula. Sites 78 and 80 are halfway to the peninsula's point. These two sites having parking pads at the road's edge, but the campsite is set up in the woods 10 yards farther from the road. At the point are eight additional sites with decks also overlooking the lake. Of those sites, sites 113, 115, and 116 offer the most unobstructed views of the lake and also have space for a large tent. The view of the lake, with its forested shoreline, is mesmerizing during the fall leaf-changing season. Area Two is shaped like a boot, and at the eastern tip of the boot's toe are sites 158 and 161. Both are spacious sites with a mix of shade and sun. These sites are out of sight of the heart of the campground, sitting peacefully at its rear.

The primitive equestrian camp sits across the lake. From US 50, follow Upp Road north 1.29 miles to trailer parking and camping on the left. Paint Creek is controlled by the U.S. Army Corps of Engineers. Visit their office located near the Paint Creek Lake Dam off of Rapid Forge Road, south of Taylor Road, for current information concerning special water releases for kayaking Paint Creek. Rock climbing is available at the spillway wall and on the Harmony Trail, both accessible from the dam and spillway parking lots.

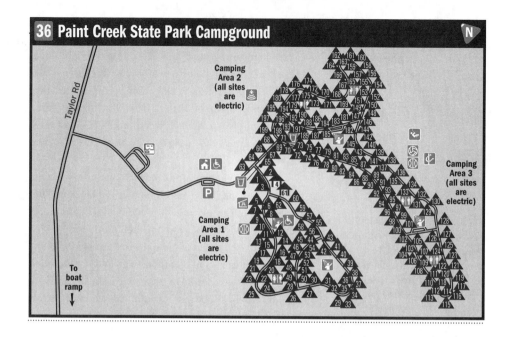

GETTING THERE

From Bainbridge, follow US 50 west for 4.44 miles to Rapid Forge Road on the right. Travel north on Rapid Forge Road for 3.7 miles to Taylor Road on the left. Follow Taylor Road west 0.71 mile to the park road on the left, and follow to the camp entrance.

GPS COORDINATES

N39°16.226'
W83°22.750'

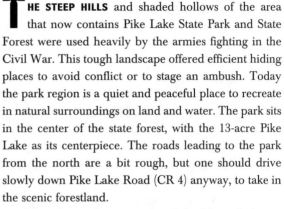

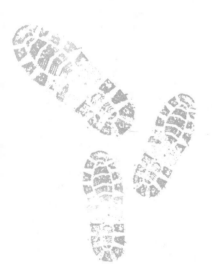

> *A quaint, out-of-the-way little park nestled among forested ridges*

THE STEEP HILLS and shaded hollows of the area that now contains Pike Lake State Park and State Forest were used heavily by the armies fighting in the Civil War. This tough landscape offered efficient hiding places to avoid conflict or to stage an ambush. Today the park region is a quiet and peaceful place to recreate in natural surroundings on land and water. The park sits in the center of state forest, with the 13-acre Pike Lake as its centerpiece. The roads leading to the park from the north are a bit rough, but one should drive slowly down Pike Lake Road (CR 4) anyway, to take in the scenic forestland.

Near the southwest corner of the lake—which was dug by hand by members of the Civilian Conservation Corps in the 1930s—is a crossroads. On the north side is the park office, with the camp store next door. The camp store has all you'll need while camping at Pike Lake, and if you didn't bring your canoe, you can rent one here. The lakeshore is just across the road to the east. To the west of the crossroad (Egypt Hollow Road) is a self-guided trail, the 0.5-mile Greenbrier Trail, on the north side of Egypt Hollow Road. On the south side of Egypt Hollow Road, opposite the Greenbrier Trail, is the 0.5-mile CCC Trail. These are pleasant, short, well-defined hikes that beckon children.

To the south of the crossroads is the campground, which lies along the base of a long ridge, amid a woodlot of medium-sized trees. These provide abundant shading during leaf season. The campground doesn't have a huge footprint, at only a quarter-mile long and an eighth of a mile wide. There are 80 sites dotted strategically throughout the rectangle, but it's not a busy place, so a quiet camp is likely here. The campground is flat—almost too flat in the center, as several sites stay moist during rains. A bulletin board with self-registration materials greets campers. Dedicated friends of the state park

RATINGS

Beauty: ☆ ☆
Privacy: ☆ ☆
Spaciousness: ☆ ☆
Quiet: ☆ ☆
Security: ☆ ☆ ☆
Cleanliness: ☆ ☆

regularly hold events open to all campers, and these are posted here. Sites 1–23 parallel Pike Lake Road and contend occasionally with traffic noise, but, again, the road is not overly traveled. As the campground's paved lane turns at the group camper's parking area, sites 24 and 25 are on the right. If the group camp is not occupied, then these two sites offer the most serenity.

North of site 25 and 20 yards beyond the turn back toward the entrance is site 57. Site 57 is spacious both in width and depth, dappled with a mix of shade and sun. Follow the lane around to site 64, which resembles site 57's layout, except with more trees. The valley floor stays a few degrees cooler, thanks to the heavy forest covering the ridges at the park's heart and the breezes blowing across the lake's surface, which funnel through the campground. Sites 66, 67, and 69 are the last of the most comfortable sites (full shade) before arriving back at the campground entrance. A footbridge crosses a 4-yard-wide creek from the campground to the dam area, which offers a picnic area.

From the dam area, a paved pathway follows the lake's western shoreline and provides fishing and easy canoe and kayak launching access. Two fishing piers jut out into the lake from this paved pathway. Anglers have a good shot at catching largemouth bass in the spring and fall, or catfish during the summer. On an island in the lake's northern tip are a swimming beach and the shower house, which are accessible by footbridge. Kayaking anglers can catch a crappie in the early spring around this bridge, to fill their skillets for a tasty camp lunch.

Pike Lake State Park is off the beaten path, and at least a dozen miles of travel are required to arrive at nearby facilities. But with several miles of well-groomed trails leading through lovely forest, and such a pretty little lake, there's plenty to see and do to fill a weekend at this park.

KEY INFORMATION

ADDRESS: 1847 Pike Lake Rd. Bainbridge, OH 45612-9640

OPERATED BY: ODNR Division of State Parks

INFORMATION: (740) 493-2212; www.dnr.state .oh.us/parks

RESERVATIONS: (866) 644-6727; www.ohio.reserve world.com

OPEN: Year-round; limited facilities in winter months; camp store closed November–March; showers closed November–May

SITES: 80 electric

EACH SITE: Picnic table, fire ring

ASSIGNMENT: Reservable sites; walk-in sites first come, first served

REGISTRATION: Self-registration station at campground entrance

FACILITIES: Latrines, water spigots, showers at beach house, camp store, laundry, sports courts, playground, swimming beach, canoe rentals, disc golf

PARKING: At each site

FEE: $21

ELEVATION: 749 feet

RESTRICTIONS: *Pets:* On leash only *Fires:* In fire ring *Alcohol:* Prohibited *Vehicles:* 2 per site *Other:* Quiet hours 10 p.m.–8 a.m.; gathering firewood prohibited; limit 6 persons per site

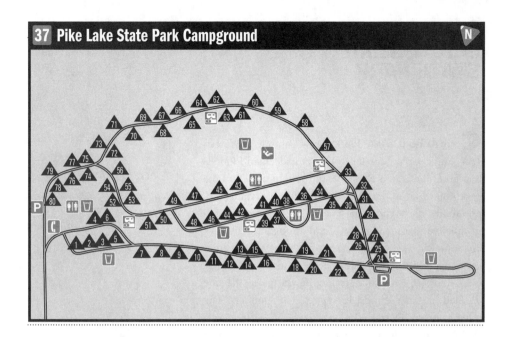

GETTING THERE

From Bainbridge, follow
CR 28 south for 3.05 miles
to CR 31 to the right. Travel
0.51 mile to CR 4, and
follow CR 4 south for 2.69
miles to the campground
entrance on the left.

GPS COORDINATES

N39°9.499'
W83°13.260'

38
SCIOTO TRAIL
STATE PARK

SCIOTO TRAIL STATE PARK sprawls among the forest-lands at the doorstep to the Appalachian foothills bordering the Scioto River. With the remoteness of the park comes an abundance of wildlife observation opportunities, throughout the year. The paved and well-maintained roads leading into, and throughout, the park are somewhat steep and curvy, but they allow campers to explore the true nature of the park and state forest. There are two campgrounds in the park; the one detailed here is the most inviting to tent campers. The other caters to RVers.

Arriving at the park's western edge on State Route 372, also named Stoney Creek Road, the first of two 15-acre lakes of the park will be on the right. If you're not paying attention, you may miss it, as it lays back in a wooded ravine 40 yards from a paved parking area that also serves a picnic shelter. Stewart Lake is accessible for fishing from its entire perimeter by following the Stewart Lake Trail. Although a kayak will have to be transported on foot to the lake for some calm paddling, the remote environment here is a treat. Don't expect to see many other paddlers on this lake because of the extra effort required to put the boat into the water.

Across the road from the Stewart Lake parking area is a similar paved parking area with a wood sign welcoming campers to the hike-in only, 18-site campground. A paved path rolls down a slight grade to the campground and is for foot traffic only. The campground sits in the bottom of a small, forested valley with a stream cutting through its center. The first sites on the right, sites 56–59, are spread out on a level, mowed lawn area with a few medium-sized trees as company. These four sites do catch some road noise from Stoney Creek Road, which is the primary thoroughfare of the park, but are perfect for a multiple family camping excursion. Site 60 is the next site on the right—it matches the first four in description

> *Scioto offers remote, dense forest with plenty of access throughout the park.*

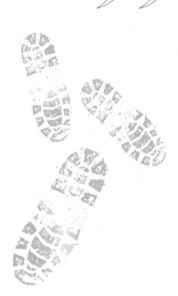

RATINGS

Beauty: ✩ ✩ ✩
Privacy: ✩ ✩ ✩
Spaciousness: ✩ ✩ ✩
Quiet: ✩ ✩ ✩
Security: ✩ ✩
Cleanliness: ✩ ✩ ✩

ADDRESS:	144 Lake Road Chillicothe, OH 45601
OPERATED BY:	ODNR Division of State Parks
INFORMATION:	(740) 887-4818); www.dnr.state .oh.us/parks
RESERVATIONS:	(866) 644-6727; www.ohio.reserve world.com
OPEN:	Year-round; limited facilities in winter
SITES:	18 hike-in, non-electric; 55 (40 electric) sites at Caldwell Lake
EACH SITE:	Picnic table, fire ring
ASSIGNMENT:	Reservable sites; walk-in sites first come, first served
REGISTRATION:	Self-registration station at camp-ground office
FACILITIES:	Latrines, water fountains, store, sports courts, play-ground, mini-golf, swimming beach, canoe rentals
PARKING:	Parking area, hike-in sites; at each site, main campground
FEE:	$23 electric; $19 nonelectric, hike-in; $2 off in winter; $1 off Sun.–Thurs.
ELEVATION:	829 feet
RESTRICTIONS:	*Pets:* On leash only *Fires:* In fire ring *Alcohol:* Prohibited *Vehicles:* 2 per site *Other:* Quiet hours 10 p.m.–8 a.m.; gathering firewood prohibited; limit 6 persons per site

but sits next to the access path to a second section of the campground.

Look for a bulletin board with park and camp rules, as well as current events, where the campground splits into two, single-file sections, at site 73. Next to the bulletin board is a water spigot. Across the paved path from the bulletin board are two latrines. The path continues up a slight grade to the last site of that line of sites, site 69. The forest climbs quickly at the rear of site 69, so expect woodland critters to drop down for a nighttime visit (nothing too big or bad, but an occasional raccoon). Head back to the split in the path and cross the small stream that flows through a culvert to reach the second row of sites.

A dozen yards beyond the stream crossing and to the right, in the middle of a 10-yard forest clearing, are sites 61 and 62. During the green season, head-high vegetation grows along the streambed and between the site rows for added privacy. In the fall, the aroma of the encroaching forest is attention-grabbing strong—a pleasant time to occupy this campground. Sites 63–68 complete the north row. These sites are the farthest from the parking area and the road (200 yards), so go straight to one of those sites for the most tranquility.

As you enter the hike-in campground pathway, a wide path through the forest will be on the left. This uphill trail (0.6 mile) leads to the fire tower and a grand view of the park. Another trail worth trekking is the Church Hollow Trail that connects to the main RV campground at Caldwell Lake. This 2-mile trail rises more than 200 feet in elevation as it explores heavy forest cover before returning to the main campground. Check out the old log church at the campground, and read the interpretive signage about the history behind it.

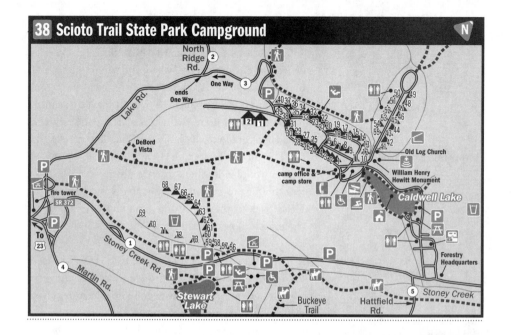

GETTING THERE

From Chillicothe, follow US 23 south for 10.98 miles to OH 372 on the left and the park entrance. Travel 1.72 miles to the primitive camping area parking on left.

GPS COORDINATES

N39°13.078'
W82°57.722'

39
SHAWNEE STATE PARK

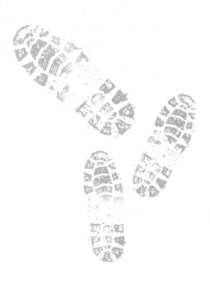

> *More than 63,000 acres of vast forest to explore—get started!*

THIS **AREA IS ONE OF** the most naturally scenic in the state, with steep hills and cut valleys that have earned Shawnee State Park and the surrounding state forest the nickname "The Little Smokies of Ohio." First-class hiking trails guide visitors to inspiring views and interactions with the vast forest. The mix of hemlock and deciduous forest that shades most of the campground presents a "mountain forest" atmosphere. The renowned Turkey Creek Nature Center, located 1 mile north of the campground on State Route 125, offers programs that are informative and entertaining for all visitors, especially young campers. Call (740) 858-6887 for the naturalist's schedule. Walking about the Shawnee State Park and forest anytime of year is a pleasurable experience, but for a wildflower show that includes rare orchids, late spring is prime time. The natural diversity displayed throughout the park and forest is abundant, warranting a multiday stay.

The campground is located between two lakes, Turkey Creek Lake and Roosevelt Lake, on the lower slope of a hill. The 107 sites here are dispersed through the woods and open areas, and up and down the slope, creating a variety of site styles at various elevations. The first sites on the right past the campground office are sites 57, 59, 61, and 63. These sit on a shelf 20 feet below the road and parking space, shaded by large trees. They are decent tent sites, but better ones exist at Shawnee State Park, if they are not occupied. The sites at the northern tip of the campground are popular with the RV owners. As the campground road turns back uphill and straightens out, site 99 is on the right. Across the road are sites 104 and 106, both set on a ledge in a woodlot.

At the southern turn of the campground's long section are sites 40 and 42. Both have a dozen wooden steps leading up from the parking space to the site. Site 38 has only six steps to climb. The forest surrounds

RATINGS

Beauty: ✩ ✩ ✩
Privacy: ✩ ✩ ✩
Spaciousness: ✩ ✩
Quiet: ✩ ✩
Security: ✩ ✩ ✩
Cleanliness: ✩ ✩ ✩

each site separately, like little barricaded forts—these are three of the quietest in the campground. Behind these sites the hill continues to rise 300 feet in elevation before reaching its peak. There are no trails through this section of the forest, so listen to the undisturbed fauna going about its business after dark for some bedtime entertainment. Following the campground road back toward the campground office, three walk-in sites lay to the right along a row of trees at the upper edge of a small swale. Sites 108–110 are complete with tent pads and a swath of lawn for the kids to burn up extra energy before making s'mores.

The block-shaped section consisting of sites 1–33 is the closest to the campground office and makes up the busiest section of the campground. A mini-golf course, amphitheater, and playground attract attention here. Traveling through the 100-yard-wide block of sites, search out site 8 at the uphill corner, as it separates itself from the pack with a few extra yards of space between neighboring sites. Also on the uphill side, but at the next corner, are sites 12–14. These sites are similar in layout and forest cover to sites 40 and 42. Of those sites, site 14 gets the nod for creating a private, forest camping experience.

A modern lodge at the park allows campers to use its swimming pool for a small fee. To find the lodge, take Forest Service Road 16 off of State Route 125, just north of the headwaters of Turkey Creek Lake. To take a walk through a deep section of the 63,000-acre state forest, jump on the 7.2-mile Shawnee State Forest Day Hike Trail. The trailhead is located on the east side of State Route 125, opposite the turn to the Turkey Creek Nature Center—follow the blue blazes. To explore the state forest from the road, try the self-guided auto tour outlined by the Division of Forestry. For a brochure and map, visit **www.ohiodnr.com** and follow the Forest links, or call (740) 858-6685.

KEY INFORMATION

ADDRESS:	4404 State Rte. 125 West Portsmouth, OH 45663
OPERATED BY:	ODNR Division of State Parks
INFORMATION:	(740) 858-4561; www.dnr.state .oh.us/parks
RESERVATIONS:	(866) 644-6727; www.ohio.reserve world.com
OPEN:	Year-round; limited facilities in winter; store closed Dec.–Mar.
SITES:	6 nonelectric; 101 electric
EACH SITE:	Picnic table, fire ring
ASSIGNMENT:	Reservable sites; walk-in sites first come, first served
REGISTRATION:	Self-registration station at campground office
FACILITIES:	Showers, flush toilets, laundry, camp store, sports courts, playground, swimming beach, boat rentals, miniature golf, nature center
PARKING:	At each site
FEE:	$24 electric; $19 nonelectric; $2 off in winter; $1 off Sunday–Thursday
ELEVATION:	717 feet
RESTRICTIONS:	*Pets:* On leash only *Fires:* In fire ring *Alcohol:* Prohibited *Vehicles:* 2 per site *Other:* Quiet hours 10 p.m.–8 a.m.; gathering firewood prohibited; limit 6 persons per site

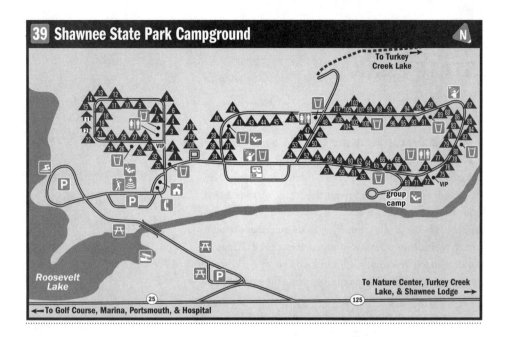

GETTING THERE

From Portsmouth, follow US 52 southwest for 6.53 miles to OH 125 on the right. Travel OH 125 for 5.36 miles to the park entrance on the left.

GPS COORDINATES

N38°43.657'
W83°10.745'

STONELICK STATE PARK

THE 200-ACRE STONELICK LAKE is a gem with clear, clean water that begs for recreation. The sights, sounds, and smells of the lake (which allows only electric motors) rise and mix with the forest scattered over Stonelick State Park, creating a naturally pleasing atmosphere. If you prefer a shot of some manmade excitement, visit Ohio's premium amusement park, Kings Island, which is less than a 30-minute drive away. You will appreciate Stonelick's welcoming, peaceful environment after a day at the park.

Camping at Stonelick is diverse; from sites at the edge of brushy habitat that supports entertaining birdlife year-round, to premium sites along the lakeshore, offering direct access to the water. The shoreline sites are labeled premium and require an extra two dollars for a (required) reservation. Because there are only nine premium sites, reserve these at least two weeks in advance. The grounds slope slightly toward the lake, with the center of the campground on a fairly even plane. The campground is mostly shaded, but not covered, by a heavy canopy from the sweet gum trees that are plentiful throughout the park. At the campground's north tip are sites 14–17, which circle a cul-de-sac. These four well-spaced sites are the most out of the way, rimmed by forest and brush. If the lakeshore sites are occupied, consider one of these.

The next cul-de-sac to the south contains four of those premium sites, each spaced from the next by 10 yards. Sites 24–27 are on the lakeshore, but the shoreline at that point is fairly brushy, with limited access for fishing or boating—but the birding opportunities are plentiful. If that circle of sites is full, try for the neighboring cul-de-sac that also sits at the water's edge, sites 28–30. These sites sit near the water level, so sliding a kayak in is easy. In fact, adjacent to site 29 is the dirt rental-boat launch point; for canoes and kayaks, a boat launch ramp

> *Fossil hunters consider Stonelick a treasure chest for rare finds.*

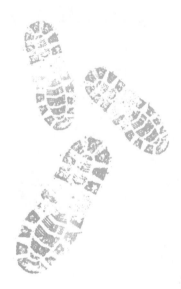

RATINGS

Beauty: ✿ ✿
Privacy: ✿ ✿
Spaciousness: ✿ ✿ ✿
Quiet: ✿ ✿
Security: ✿ ✿ ✿
Cleanliness: ✿ ✿ ✿

KEY INFORMATION

ADDRESS: 2895 Lake Drive Pleasant Plain, OH 45162

OPERATED BY: ODNR Division of State Parks

INFORMATION: (513) 625-6593; www.dnr.state .oh.us/parks

RESERVATIONS: (866) 644-6727; www.ohio.reserve world.com

OPEN: Year-round; limited facilities in winter; store and heated showers closed Dec.–Mar.

SITES: 6 nonelectric; 108 electric

EACH SITE: Picnic table, fire ring

ASSIGNMENT: Reservable sites; walk-in sites first come, first served

REGISTRATION: Self-registration station at campground office

FACILITIES: Showers, flush toilets, laundry, camp store, sports courts, playground, swimming beach, boat rentals, bike rentals

PARKING: At each site

FEE: $20 nonelectric; $24 electric; $2 off in winter; $1 off Sunday–Thursday

ELEVATION: 902 feet

RESTRICTIONS: *Pets:* On leash only *Fires:* In fire ring *Alcohol:* Prohibited *Vehicles:* 2 per site *Other:* Quiet hours 10 p.m.–7 a.m.; gathering firewood prohibited; limit 6 persons per site; no parking on grass

is located off of State Route 727, on the lake's west side. Site 29 begs for a couple of chairs positioned at the water's edge after dinner, to release any stress while observing a sunset over the lake.

The next cul-de-sac to the south holds the nonelectric sites, sites 33–39. Of those sites, sites 34 and 35 offer views of the lake but no direct access. The abundance of space at those sites, each about 15 yards by 15 yards, creates quiet campsites, with a pretty lake to admire. This section may be quietest for tent campers because of the abundant space and the brushy screen between the neighboring sites.

The main and central loop of the campground is shaped like a peanut, with two premium sites (53 and 55) sitting at the western edge. Sites 53 and 55 have lake views, not lake access, as a steep, brush-covered slope several yards in length keeps campers at bay. The higher vantage point here, however, offers a panoramic view. The center of the peanut is filled with sites that feel like being in a neighborhood, each site open to the next. Sprouting off of the peanut section and ending at a cul-de-sac are sites 68–86. At the outer edge of this cul-de-sac is site 76, which sits above a southern cove of the lake but only offers lake views when the trees are bare. The last and southernmost campground section includes sites 90–113. These are the first seen upon entering the campground on the left and fill the bill of most RVers—flat, with no low branches to obstruct awnings.

The bedrock that lies under Stonelick raised up near the earth's surface as the Appalachian Mountains were created thousands of years ago. That fact has drawn fossil hunters to the region for centuries. Fossils of the rarest form and variety are still collected today throughout southwestern Ohio, but especially in the region that includes Stonelick State Park. Designated areas are open to fossil collecting; call the park office at (513) 734-4323 to access permitted locations.

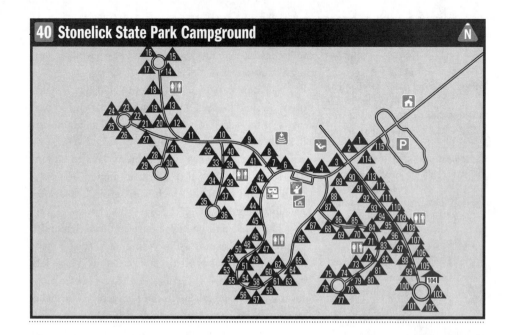

GETTING THERE

From Blanchester, travel 5.68 miles southwest on OH 133 to Edenton. Follow OH 727 southwest 2.39 miles to Lake Drive on the left. Travel 2.12 miles on Lake Road to the campground entrance.

GPS COORDINATES

N39°13.024'
W84°3.527'

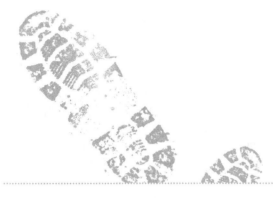

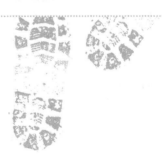

CENTRAL

A.W. MARION STATE PARK

A.W. **MARION STATE PARK** and its pleasing little lake are testaments to the adage that good things come in small packages. The park covers 309 land acres and its star feature—Hargus Lake— takes up half of that space, at 145 acres. The lake is a kettle lake, created by a piece of glacier melting, and the vegetation that grows in and around the lake today are the ancestors of the seeds gathered and left by the glacier. The park's fertile soils continue annually to produce some of the state's most dazzling wildflowers. To witness the park's botanical diversity, cinch up your boot strings and set out on the 5-mile Hargus Lake Perimeter Trail that begins at the campground.

Hargus Lake is best explored by boat, which you can rent at the clean and well-stocked little marina on the west shore, across the lake from the campground. The lake has an electric motors–only restriction, so there are no wakes to worry about. The lake was drained in the early 1980s, when it received fish habitat improvements and was restocked. There are three small islands and two peninsulas to explore. One lap around serene Hargus Lake via canoe or kayak will leave you wanting more.

The park's isolated campground sprawls out on top of a ridge, 50 feet higher in elevation than Hargus Lake. During the summer, a view of the lake doesn't exist, but in the autumn when the leaves fall from the oaks standing throughout the campground, a scenic shot of the lake is revealed. The camping fun begins at the end of a dead-end road. The campground's small size forced planners to squeeze as many sites onto the property as possible. The first sites on the right when entering the campground are the tightest, so drive past those around the long loop and watch for site 56 on the right. Site 56 has more elbow room than the previous ones, and it sports a tent pad and lantern holder as well. Site 57 is similar, and they both sit at the edge of a hollow that leads to the lake.

> *Can't get enough of this small, tranquil lake*

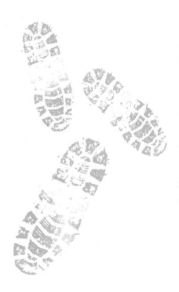

RATINGS

Beauty: ✩ ✩
Privacy: ✩ ✩
Spaciousness: ✩ ✩
Quiet: ✩ ✩
Security: ✩ ✩ ✩
Cleanliness: ✩ ✩

KEY INFORMATION

ADDRESS: 7317 Warner-
Huffer Road
Circleville, OH
43113

OPERATED BY: ODNR Division of
State Parks

INFORMATION: (740) 869-3124;
www.dnr.state
.oh.us/parks

RESERVATIONS: (866) 644-6727;
www.ohio.reserve
world.com

OPEN: Closed Nov.–Mar.

SITES: 29 nonelectric;
29 electric

EACH SITE: Fire ring, picnic
table

ASSIGNMENT: Reservable sites;
walk-in sites first
come, first served

REGISTRATION: Self-registration at
campground
entrance

FACILITIES: Latrines, playground, amphithe-
atre, pay phone;
sports courts, boat
rentals

PARKING: At each site

FEE: $19 nonelectric;
$23 electric; $1 off
Sun.–Thurs.; $2 off
in winter

ELEVATION: 893 feet

RESTRICTIONS: *Pets:* Must be on
leash; two pets per
site maximum
Fires: In fire ring
Alcohol: Prohibited
Vehicles: Must fit on
paved pad; extra
vehicles to be
parked in lot near
park office
Other: Quiet hours
10 p.m.–8 a.m.;
gathering firewood
prohibited; limit 6
persons per site

Back near the entrance is a small semi-loop with sites 17–27. These sites also offer an extra few feet to spread out. Site 23 has the Hargus Lake Perimeter Trail pass through its edge, which may bring some visitors too close for comfort. Instead, try site 21 for more privacy. Sites 19 and 22 are inside the loop and are good second choices because they are still several yards away from the campground's main road. The last set of sites from which to choose sits in a small loop to the east of the entrance. Site 8 offers the most space and rests at the campground's outer edge.

The Stages Pond State Nature Preserve north of A.W. Marion State Park is worth a visit. Return to Ringold Southern Road and head north to Stout Road. Turn left on Stout and travel to OH 188. Drive southwest on OH 188 and take the first right, Winchester Road. Go north 2 miles to Hagerty Road and turn left. The nature preserve will be on the right in 2.21 miles. Stages Pond is another kettle lake viewed from maintained trails. During the spring and fall, the lake is a refuge for migrating waterfowl, some of which are rare in Ohio, such as the greater white-fronted goose (aka specklebelly). During the summer, the calls and songs of various species of shorebirds echo out across the nature preserve.

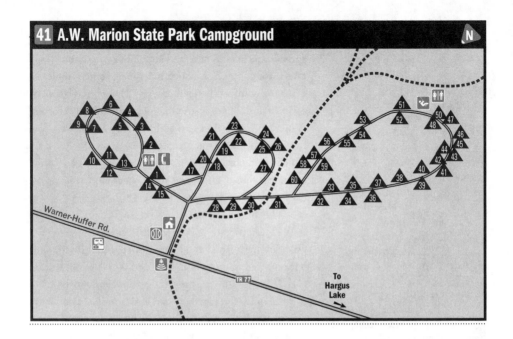

Warner-Huffer Rd.

TR 77

To
Hargus
Lake

GETTING THERE

From Circleville, follow
OH 22 east for 3.9 miles to
Ringold Southern Road
(TR 42). Turn left and travel
0.85 mile north to Warner-
Huffer Road (TR 77) on the
left. Travel west 0.44 mile to
the campground entrance
on the left.

GPS COORDINATES

N39°38.073'
W82°52.931'

42
DELAWARE STATE PARK

A lake built to control flooding is now flooded with recreation.

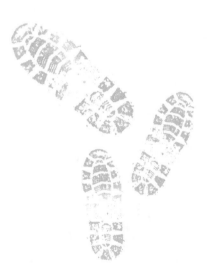

THE **US ARMY CORPS OF ENGINEERS** constructed the Delaware Lake in 1948 for flood control, and it has been a popular recreation destination ever since. Located fewer than 30 miles from the state's capitol, the Delaware State Park, with its mix of forest and meadows, is a popular park. The mixed forest on the lake's east side is a managed wildlife area, primarily used for hunting. But when hunting season is closed, the food plots and other conservational practices here are great for wildlife viewing. Seven miles south of the town of Delaware, on the busy US Route 23 and then right on Home Road, sit the Olentangy Caverns. For less than $10, you can take a guided tour of the caves that were once an important asset for the Delaware Indians.

The 211 campsites in the park are split into four clusters along the lake's west side. The lake is accessible by foot via designated hiking trails from a few of the sites, and there are tie-ups for boaters willing to leave their boats unattended. The clusters of campsites, named numbered "areas," are arranged like five-petal flowers. Each cluster contains 50 sites, with 10 sites per branch. The first right past the campground office and store leads to Area Four and passes the park road (remember the flower stem?) to Area Three on the way.

In the center of each cluster is a shower house with flush toilets and a laundry room. Area Four has sites 1–50. The first branch (or petal) opens with sites 1 and 2, both shaded and with no neighbors across the lane. Sites 12 and 13 sit in the second branch and are set back in a pocket in the woods. The third branch offers site 27, among a mix of deciduous trees. Access to the 1.5-mile Briarpatch Trail passes behind site 27. The trail winds through a mix of young forest, meadows, and a couple of ponds hidden in the woods. The 20 sites in the fourth and fifth branches of Area Four are better left for RVs.

RATINGS

Beauty: ☆ ☆
Privacy: ☆ ☆
Spaciousness: ☆ ☆
Quiet: ☆ ☆
Security: ☆ ☆ ☆
Cleanliness: ☆ ☆ ☆

Area Three can be bypassed for tent camping—this cluster is also more attractive to RVers. Return to the lane you came in on, Park Road 27, turn right, and travel approximately 0.40 mile to Area Two. Pass up the first branch, consisting of sites 101–111, and drive into the second branch to site 113 on the right. It's a shaded site not far from the shower house and bathroom, yet far enough to enjoy some peaceful camping. The third branch has the dandy site 128. From this site you can see the lake and be on the Big Foot Trail that passes between the site and the shoreline en route to the Fisherman's Trail that heads to a quiet lake cove.

If the popular site 128 is taken, slide up the fourth branch that includes sites 134–145. All ten of these sites offer camping under large maple trees standing up and down the branch lane, and the sites are staggered from each other to reduce the "curious neighbor syndrome." Up the fifth branch, sites 155 and 156 are the best of the branch, also with a staggered position and a thick vegetation screen between them.

Leave Area Two and drive north on Park Road 27 for approximately 0.75 mile to Area One—the farthest from the campground entrance, which weeds out most RVers, and is home to two of the best branches of the campground. Area One also has the most dense forest surrounding and jutting into the campsites. The first branch has sites 158–166. Site 160 spreads out under a mature oak. Site 163 is a deep site in a group of young trees. The second branch offers site 180, a wider site for a couple of tents. Skip the third branch of sites 181–191, unless you prefer wide-open yard camping. The fourth branch extends toward the lake, which is only a short walk through the forest. The forest neighbors sites 195 and 196, with site 197 completing the trifecta—all three are steps from a trail leading to another set of boat tie-ups.

The meadows throughout the park are spotted with bird boxes attached to skinny posts. These comprise a well-thought-out and managed insect control plan. The nesting boxes, placed in a grid, 25 feet apart, attract breeding tree swallows. The tree swallows are insect-eating machines, swooping over open wetlands and marshes, catching flies and mosquitoes to feed their

KEY INFORMATION

ADDRESS: 5202 US 23 N. Delaware, OH 43015

OPERATED BY: ODNR Division of State Parks

INFORMATION: (740) 363-4561; www.dnr.state .oh.us/parks

RESERVATIONS: (866) 644-6727; www.ohio.reserve world.com

OPEN: Year-round; store closed Nov.–Mar.; showers closed Dec.–Mar.

SITES: 211 electric

EACH SITE: Picnic table, fire ring

ASSIGNMENT: Reservable sites; walk-in sites first come, first served

REGISTRATION: Self-registration station at campground office if office is closed

FACILITIES: Showers, flush toilets, laundry, camp store, game room, boat launch ramp, boat rentals, bike rentals, disc golf, swimming beach

PARKING: At each site

FEE: $27

ELEVATION: 953 feet

RESTRICTIONS: *Pets:* On leash only
Fires: In fire ring
Alcohol: Prohibited
Vehicles: 2 per site, boat trailers count as one
Other: Quiet hours 10 p.m.–8 a.m.; gathering firewood prohibited; limit 6 persons per site; 3 tents maximum per site

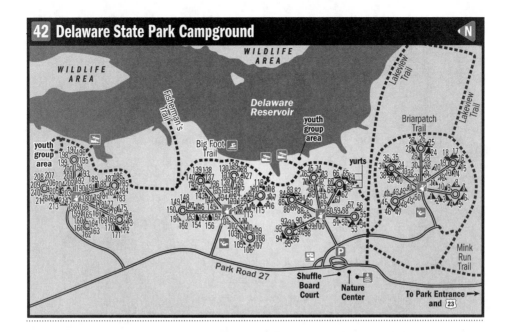

GETTING THERE

From Delaware, travel north on US 23 for 5.82 miles to the park entrance on the right. Follow signage to the campground.

young. The adult tree swallow can feed its babies up to 6,000 insects per day—an impressively efficient insect control system.

GPS COORDINATES

N40°23.73'
W83°3.74'

43
DILLON
STATE PARK

DILLON STATE PARK is a wonderful example of the evidence of the progress of transportation in America. The Licking River, once a primary travel route for Native Americans, leads to the larger Muskingum River running through downtown Zanesville and cuts the 2,285–acre state park in half. Today Dillon Dam, built in 1961, slows the Licking River for flood control, and the river is a favorite of avid canoers. Eight miles northeast of the park is the Blackhand Gorge State Nature Preserve outside of Toboso, where you can see remnants of the Ohio-Erie Canal System. Canal towpaths and locks can be seen from a 4-mile paved hike and bike trail that follows the Licking River through the pristine gorge. Vistas from the steep riverbank offer a peaceful break to soak up the sights of the river's sandstone cliffs and the sounds of birds singing and flittering about the tree canopy. An interurban railroad connected Zanesville to Newark before traveling on to Columbus by following the Licking River through the Dillon region and the Blackhand Gorge. The Old National Road passes through Zanesville and crosses the Y-Bridge—a unique and historic bridge built in the shape its name implies, crossing the confluence of the Licking and Muskingum rivers. Don't be alarmed if you ask for directions from a local resident and they tell you to take a right or a left in the middle of the bridge. The Muskingum River was a major steamboat route that allowed for the delivery of supplies to the growing settlements in east central Ohio.

Camping at Dillon State Park puts visitors between Zanesville and Newark, both of which offer natural and cultural history. Watch for members of the park's abundant deer population—they do not hesitate to form groups near the park roads. After passing the campground check station, take a right at the intersection. You will pass the shower house on the hill on the left. As you reach the left bend in the road, the 12 tent sites (sites

> *Soak up natural and cultural history at Dillon State Park.*

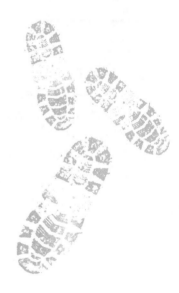

RATINGS

Beauty: ✿ ✿
Privacy: ✿
Spaciousness: ✿ ✿
Quiet: ✿ ✿
Security: ✿ ✿ ✿ ✿
Cleanliness: ✿ ✿ ✿

ADDRESS: 5265 Dillon Hills Drive, Nashport, OH 43830-9568

OPERATED BY: ODNR Division of Parks

INFORMATION: (740) 453-4377; www.dnr.state .oh.us/parks

RESERVATIONS: (866) 644-6727; www.ohio.reserve world.com

OPEN: Year-round

SITES: 183 electric, 12 nonelectric

EACH SITE: Picnic table, fire ring

ASSIGNMENT: Reservable sites; walk-in sites first come, first served

REGISTRATION: At camp office; self-registration station in front of camp office

FACILITIES: Store, showers, toilets, laundry, pay phone, playground, sports courts, nature center, boat ramp, archery range

PARKING: At each site, except tent-only sites have parking area

FEE: $24 electric, $18 nonelectric

ELEVATION: 945 feet

RESTRICTIONS: *Pets:* At all sites except 1–32
Fires: In fire ring
Alcohol: Prohibited
Vehicles: 2 per site if tent camping, 1 per site if RV on site
Other: Quiet hours 10 p.m.–8 a.m.; gathering firewood prohibited; 14-day stay limit; limit 6 persons per site

184–195) sit on the rise to your left, and their parking area is then on both sides of the road. The mowed hill on the right is a sledding hill. A slight uphill walk from the parking area is required, but a bark mulch pathway keeps it skid-free. The sites spread out evenly throughout a wood lot surrounded on three sides by the campground road that you came in on, as it winds its way to the electric sites that regularly host RVers. The security at Dillon is top-notch, and the speed limit is enforced sternly—so although the campground road passes the tent area, drivers drive by in a quiet, slow manner.

The wood lot slopes slightly toward the parking area, but this is not a problem for tent pitching. Site 189 is the farthest from the parking area and adjoining tent sites, earning this campground's best tent-site designation. A backdrop of brush curtains off any commotion coming from the RV sites over the ridge. All of the tent sites have a view (sites 185–189 have the best) of the sledding hill that is also a wildlife viewing area, flanked by forest on both sides. Speaking of wildlife, keep your snacks off the picnic table, as the healthy population of squirrels will sneak a taste when your back is turned. A restroom is accessible by taking a 20-yard walk across the campground road. The primary sites are busy through the summer with RVing families, but those sites are plenty spacious for big tenting excursions as well.

The Dillon region attracts sportsmen during the hunting seasons because of the expansive wildlife area that sprawls out and joins Dillon State Park's northern boundary, flanking the southbound-flowing Licking River. A sportsman's area is located on Pleasant Valley Road, which is located on the left after driving 5.48 miles north on OH 146 from the intersection of OH 146 and Clay Littick Drive. The sportsman's area has a 100-yard rifle range and a 25-yard pistol range. Back at the state park, an archery range is located at the bottom of the sledding hill. Sanctioned mountain bike racers visit Dillon State Park's 12-mile bike course, deemed one of the most challenging in the state. The 1,560-acre Dillon Lake is available for unlimited horsepower boating.

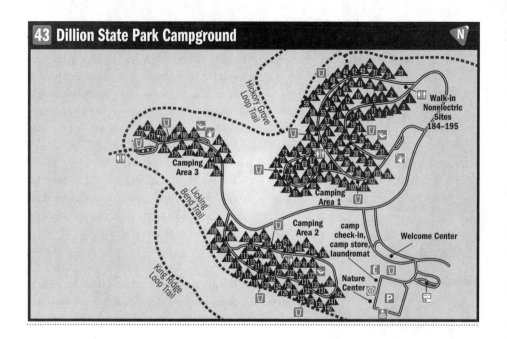

GETTING THERE

From I-70 Exit 153 in Zanesville, go north on Blue Avenue for 0.37 mile to OH 146. Turn left and travel 7.47 miles to CR 708 (Clay Littick Drive) on the left and follow for 1.61 miles to the campground entrance on the right.

GPS COORDINATES

N40°0.643'
W82°6.257'

44
ELLIS LOCK #11 AT MUSKINGUM RIVER PARKWAY STATE PARK

Fish with the eagles at this riverfront camp.

TEN LOCKS make the Muskingum River navigable from Marietta to Dresden, a 112-mile boat ride. The hand-operated locks are more than 150 years old, and all but one are still working. The one temporarily not working happens to be at this riverside campground. Because of the locks and their historical status, the Muskingum River Parkway is on the National Register of Historical Places. Of the ten locks (all have a park setting), there are two with campgrounds: one at Lock #5, for boaters only; the other is Lock #11, about 7 miles north of Zanesville, just south of Dresden. The river can be enjoyed without a boat, with the campground providing ample access to the riverbank. Huge shovelhead catfish are the stars of the gamefish in the Muskingum River—catfish the size of a small child are commonly caught here. The river's wildlife can also be enjoyed from the bench near the upriver side of the lock. For the last few years, eagles have nested less than a half mile from the campground. They are spotted occasionally feeding on shad or sitting on a high branch, looking grand.

The campground lies on approximately one acre of nearly level river frontage. A horseshoe-shaped, paved lane enters the camping area near the lock on the right, with a restroom and drinking water–supply on the left. Sites 1–6 are on the river, with plenty of space to spread out the folding chairs and take in the river scene. Sites 1 and 2 have the lock's upper retaining wall at their edge. Sites 3–6 have no wall, but the slope from the sites to the river is steep and not safe for swimming or wading, with the entrance to the lock so close. There is no safety railing along the lock wall, so it's crucial that kids are kept a safe distance from the edge. Sites 1 and 3 each have a large tree that provides shade throughout the day. Across the lane, the camp host occupies site 20. Sites 18 and 19 join site 20 in a row parallel to the river. On around the horseshoe-shaped lane, sites 7 and

RATINGS

Beauty: ✿ ✿
Privacy: ✿ ✿
Spaciousness: ✿ ✿
Quiet: ✿ ✿
Security: ✿
Cleanliness: ✿ ✿

8 on the right are against a wall of woodland/brush mix. Behind that overgrown mix are ATV trails that are not open to the public. Sites 9–12 are farthest from the river, and their back sides have a wooden fence between the parkway campground and a small private campground. A few small trees are scattered about the campground but offer little shade, except for the two mature trees.

Powelson Wildlife Area is a couple of miles west of the campground. This 2,775-acre wildlife area lies between OH 60 and the Muskingum River. As with many of the modern wildlife areas in eastern and southeastern Ohio, they are the result of strict reclamation requirements following mining that stripped the land's surface during the 1940s. The township roads that course through Powelson provide access for hunting, fishing, and hiking. Several remote ponds that hold healthy largemouth bass are pleasant destinations for the angler or day hiker feeling the need for a bit of adventure without trails. Keep an eye out for small remnants of abandoned homesteads, such as cut sandstone foundations, cast-iron cooking pots peeking up from the leafy forest floor, and even the occasional tombstone.

KEY INFORMATION

ADDRESS:	1390 Ellis Dam Road Zanesville, OH 43701
OPERATED BY:	ODNR Division of Parks
INFORMATION:	(740) 453-4377 (Dillon State Park handles this park's calls); www.dnr.state.oh.us/parks
RESERVATIONS:	(866) 644-6727; www.ohio.reserveworld.com
OPEN:	April–November
SITES:	20 nonelectric
EACH SITE:	Picnic table, fire ring
ASSIGNMENT:	Reservable sites; walk-in sites first come, first served
REGISTRATION:	At self-registration station at campground entrance
FACILITIES:	Latrine, drinking water spigot on rear of latrine building, boat ramp
PARKING:	At each site
FEE:	$16
ELEVATION:	714 feet
RESTRICTIONS:	*Pets:* Allowed but must be kept on leash *Fires:* In fire ring *Alcohol:* Prohibited *Vehicles:* 1 per site, parking lot available *Other:* Quiet hours 10 p.m.–8 a.m.; gathering firewood prohibited; 14-day stay limit; not more than 6 persons per site; major supplies available in Zanesville

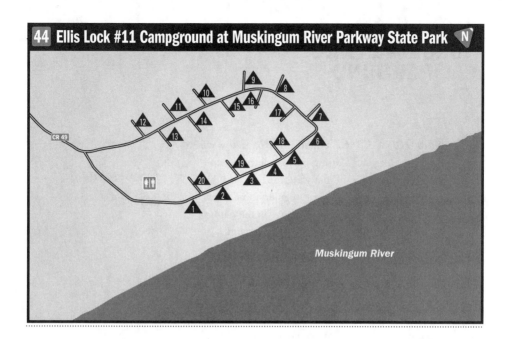

GETTING THERE

From OH 60, 6.6 miles north of Zanesville, turn east onto Richvale Road and travel 2.37 miles to Friendly Hills Road on the left. Drive 2 miles to Ellis Dam Road on the right and follow it 0.88 mile to the campground and park.

GPS COORDINATES

N40°2.645'
W81°58.671'

KOKOSING LAKE CAMPGROUND

DRIVING ALONG **CR 6,** Waterford Road, toward Kokosing Lake and Campground, you may experience flyovers from the multiple waterfowl species that visit the lake—either migrating or regular inhabitants. The 154-acre lake is not deep, but it's huge in the natural splendor that surrounds it and its fine campground. The U.S. Army Corps of Engineers constructed the Kokosing Dam in 1972 for flood control. The dammed water is now home to several species of gamefish and wildlife that inhabit the surrounding Kokosing Wildlife Area. Kayaking or canoeing from the campground across the lake to the northeast leads to an ice-cream-cone–shaped island. The island is covered in brush, as is the lake's shoreline on the side of the island farthest from the campground. Between the island and the shoreline is a quiet and out-of-sight portion of the lake that should be paddlers' first stop. Slowly paddling around the island, allowing the kayak to glide, will allow the wildlife at the water's edge to be approached at a close distance. If a watercraft is not on your trip's packing list, don't fret—most of the lake can be explored with a quality pair of binoculars or telephoto camera lens.

This campground is one of the nicest in the state. Even though RVs are common in the primary sector (there is a tent section), the tranquil, lakeside camping mood is strong there. Of the 46 sites, 17 of them—including the 4 tent sites—are on the lake's edge with great views of the sunrise and sunset over the water. After entering the campground, take the lane straight ahead and follow it past the restroom on the left—which also has a drinking water–spigot and drinking fountain in front of it—to find the tent sites, 43–46. You must walk to these four sites, but inquire with the camp office about tent site designated parking. Site 43 will be partially shaded in the morning hours but in full sun the rest of the day. The other three tent sites are in

> *Lakeside camping at its best*

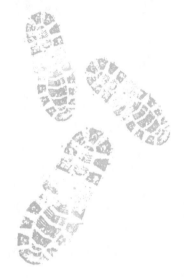

RATINGS

Beauty: ✩ ✩ ✩
Privacy: ✩ ✩ ✩
Spaciousness: ✩ ✩ ✩
Quiet: ✩ ✩
Security: ✩ ✩ ✩
Cleanliness: ✩ ✩ ✩

ADDRESS: 18350 Waterford Road Fredericktown, OH 43019

OPERATED BY: Muskingum Watershed Conservancy District

INFORMATION: (740) 694-1900 reaches camp office in season; (419) 368-6885; www.mwcd.org

RESERVATIONS: First come, first served

OPEN: May–September

SITES: 46

EACH SITE: Picnic table, fire ring

ASSIGNMENT: First come, first served

REGISTRATION: At camp office at campground entrance

FACILITIES: Showers, flush toilets and latrine, drinking water; playground, direct access to the lake, boat ramp

PARKING: At each site, except for tent sites

FEE: $23

ELEVATION: 1,136 feet

RESTRICTIONS: *Pets:* On leash only in designated areas *Fires:* In fire ring *Alcohol:* None publicly consumed or displayed *Vehicles:* 1 per site *Other:* Sites registered to campers age 18 and older; quiet hours 11 p.m.–7 a.m.; ice available at camp store; major supplies available in Mt. Vernon

full sun all day, with access to the lake only a few steps away. The tent section is like setting up camp in a wide, nicely mowed backyard, except this yard has a lake adjacent. The shoreline is gravel, which is easy on the feet if a few minutes of wading are needed to cool off. A second drinking water–spigot is located in the center of the loop, surrounded by sites near the tent section. These loop sites are shaded at least half the day and sit off the water but close enough to see the lake.

Back in the campground's primary section sit four lakeside sites attractive to any camper. Site 15 is shaded nearly all day and offers plenty of space. Site 18 offers the most privacy and has an inlet off the lake, separating it from site 20. Site 20 is also a spacious, shady site. Site 22 gets the nod for the best of this group. It has a large, level (as is most of the campground) area to accommodate large tents and shares occupancy with a shade-giving sycamore. The site is out on a point in the lake where good fishing can be had not far from shore, as the water depth drops off quickly to the east. A modern shower house is positioned on a hill above the campground, an easy stroll from all sites.

There are no established hiking trails here, but less than a half mile back on Waterford Road the Kokosing Dam is accessible. A parking area and bulletin board are available for visitors at the end of a short dam access road. Hikers often utilize this parking area for day hiking the Kokosing Wildlife Area, a mix of forest and fields. The fields are managed as food sources for wildlife. Spending several minutes hiking through the diverse natural enhancements, you will soon discover you are not alone. Depending on the season, pause occasionally and see how many different subspecies of butterflies you can count. Or sit high on the dam and take in the lake view below. And that tent off to the left, at the tip of the campground—that may be yours.

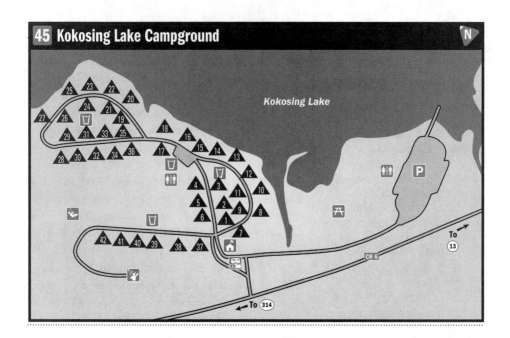

Kokosing Lake

To 13

CR 6

To 314

GETTING THERE

From OH 13 northwest of
Fredericktown, drive west
on CR 6 for 1.9 miles to the
campground entrance on
the right.

GPS COORDINATES

N40°30.379'
W82°35.173'

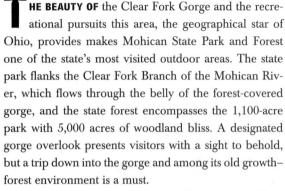

A gorge, rich forest, clear river, and campsites are all here to enjoy.

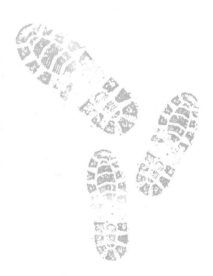

THE BEAUTY OF the Clear Fork Gorge and the recreational pursuits this area, the geographical star of Ohio, provides makes Mohican State Park and Forest one of the state's most visited outdoor areas. The state park flanks the Clear Fork Branch of the Mohican River, which flows through the belly of the forest-covered gorge, and the state forest encompasses the 1,100-acre park with 5,000 acres of woodland bliss. A designated gorge overlook presents visitors with a sight to behold, but a trip down into the gorge and among its old growth–forest environment is a must.

The Mohican State Park and Forest Region host three campground systems. The most popular is the Class A Area Campground, which caters primarily to RVers. A short drive deeper into the park, you will find the Class B Area Campground, a.k.a. Hemlock Grove Campground, a primitive campground. Located on the north central ridge above both camping areas A and B are three Park and Pack Sites managed by the ODNR's Division of Forestry.

The Class A Campground is a bustling place throughout the summer camping season. Families preferring the comforts of RVs fill this campground, which creates a friendly neighborhood atmosphere. But tucked away in the southwest corner of this busy campground are ten nonelectric sites that are accessed by foot only. After passing through the main campground gate and registration station, take the first left. After making that left, on the left is parking for the ten walk-in sites. Across from this parking lot is a restroom, and a few steps to the left of the restroom is a source for potable water.

From the parking area, cross the short footbridge over a drainage ditch to find sites 1 thru 4 spread from left to right. These four sites sit on mowed cutouts among a mix of short ornamental shrubs and smaller deciduous trees—plenty of shade and 40 yards from the river. The

RATINGS

Beauty: ✩ ✩ ✩ ✩
Privacy: ✩ ✩ ✩
Spaciousness: ✩ ✩ ✩
Quiet: ✩ ✩ ✩
Security: ✩ ✩
Cleanliness: ✩ ✩

more preferred sites of the group are 5–10, which sit only a few steps from water. These sites are normally full during summer weekends, but springtime river paddlers and autumn foliage fans will find ample vacancy. Large sycamores intermixed with additional tall trees provide cool camping along the river. Site 10 receives the least amount of passing foot traffic.

The Class B Campground entrance is near one of the Mohican Region's most visited landmarks—a covered bridge over the Clear Fork River. To access the campground, you must drive through Hemlock Grove Picnic Area, just east of the bridge. A self-registration kiosk welcomes campers to the 25-site, nonelectric campground. The campground road follows the river, with all campsites on the opposite side of the road, but along the road's edge. Potable water and pit latrines are available across from site 18, as is a fishing access and parking point. The trout fishing here is considered as good as it gets in Ohio. During early and late seasons, the campsites here are utilized regularly by anglers. The last site on the dead-end road, site 25, provides the most privacy. The Hemlock Gorge hiking trail connects the Class B Area to the Class A Area by following a pleasing stroll along one of Ohio's Scenic Rivers. Keep in mind that this stretch of river gets a steady stream of autos touring the gorge, especially during weekends, so expect to deal with sightseers.

For campers wanting to get their fill of deep woods camping without neighbors, the Mohican State Forest's Park and Pack Sites fill the bill. There are ten of these remote campsites throughout the Mohican State Forest. Sites 1–7 cater to equestrians and sit along popular bridle trails. Sites 8, 9, and 10 are situated on Hickory Ridge, which runs along the north central border of the Mohican State Forest. With access to these three sites by mountain bike or on foot only, these are premium tent-camping targets (a fire ring is the only item provided). A gravel road leads to a small parking area (patrolled by law enforcement), with signage posted there that points the way to each site.

Site 8 is a 10-minute casual walk from the parking area (even with a pack of gear). Keep watch for the occasional, fast-moving mountain biker, as the multiuse trail

KEY INFORMATION

ADDRESS:	3116 State Route 3 Loudonville, OH 44842
OPERATED BY:	ODNR Division of State Parks
INFORMATION:	(419) 994-5125; www.dnr.state .oh.us/parks
RESERVATIONS:	(866) 644-6727; www.ohio.reserve world.com
OPEN:	Year-round; limited facilities in winter
SITES:	189
EACH SITE:	Picnic table, fire ring
ASSIGNMENT:	Reservable sites; walk-in sites first come, first served (entire Class B Area included)
REGISTRATION:	At campground office; self-register at office if closed
FACILITIES:	Showers, flush toilets, latrines, laundry, pay phone, pool, playground, sports courts, canoe launch, commissary, nature center
PARKING:	At each site
FEE:	$31 electric; $21 nonelectric; $1 off Sun.–Thurs.; $2 off in winter
ELEVATION:	928 feet
RESTRICTIONS:	*Pets:* On leash only *Fires:* In fire ring *Alcohol:* Prohibited *Vehicles:* 2 per site *Other:* Quiet hours 10 p.m.–8 a.m.; gathering firewood prohibited; must pay entry fee; limit 6 persons per site

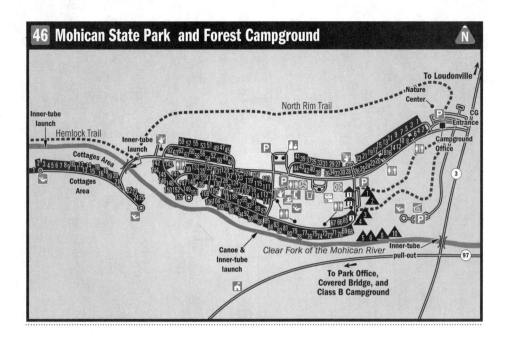

GETTING THERE

From Loudonville, take OH 3 south 2.31 miles to the Mohican State Park entrance. Class A Area camping is on the right through the main entrance. To access Class B Area camping, continue on OH 3 past the main entrance 0.24 mile to OH 97 on right. Take OH 97, 2.95 miles to park road (signage posted) on right. Follow to the left 1.25 miles to the campground once across the covered bridge. For Mohican State Forest camping, from the same covered bridge, continue on park road 1.1 miles to CR 939. Travel north 0.58 mile to CR3006, turn right, and go 0.21 mile to TR 3006. Follow TR 3006 0.93 mile to camper parking on the right, at the end of the dead-end road.

is a favorite with cyclists. Site 8 is similar to the other two—laid out on a heavily forested finger ridge, near the rim of the river gorge—but it offers the least amount of view and space. Site 9 is less crowded with smaller trees and ground brush, but it is a 15-minute walk from the car. Site 10 requires the longest trek, 20 minutes, but it's worth the extra effort as the remoteness is best felt here. These sites lead campers through rich forests that host seldom-seen flora and fauna, such as the wild blue phlox blooming in the spring.

Note: The Park and Pack sites are free, but you must self-register.

GPS COORDINATES

CLASS A AREA :	STATE FOREST SITES 8-10:
N40°36.580' W82°15.450'	N40°37.216' W82°17.109'
CLASS B AREA: N40°36.819' W82°18.983'	

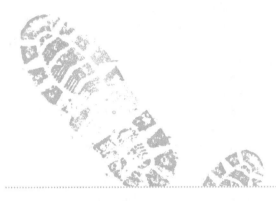

LAKE ERIE REGION

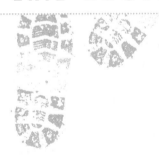

EAST HARBOR STATE PARK

THE SHORES OF WESTERN Lake Erie continue to be a serious vacation destination. This is true for families and adventurous individuals alike. Seven million people visit the great lake each year, but still there are quiet places to take in an abundance of natural beauty and interaction. East Harbor State Park is one of those places. East Harbor State Park is on the east side of the Catawba peninsula and on the western shore of East Harbor. The park is surrounded by vacation activities such as fishing Lake Erie and the harbors, wildlife-watching, and sightseeing. Inside the park is the Ohio State Park System's largest campground. Even so, tent campers have their own place where RVs don't tread, although the RVs are within sight.

Campground sections B, C, and E cater to RVs of every size. A few tents are regularly sprinkled among them, but for the serious tent camper, sections A and D (G is a group section) are quietly positioned in forested settings. Section A is the largest of the tent-site sections and surrounds a wide-open playing field and playground area. Sites A1–A89 line both sides of several paved roads that create a gridlike layout. Sites A90–A114 line the outer perimeter of section A; shade covers the rear of each site, and some of these sites have total shade. Sites A116–A140 are in full shade, and sites A141–A179 are open to the sun. Sites A79–A89 are at the back side of section A and are the most quiet sites away from other section A campers and campground traffic rolling in and out of sections B and A.

Section D, located on the opposite side of the campground from section A, is tucked away in a small wooded grove and offers 20 sites. Sites D1–D16 are comfortable for tent campers with efficient tent-pitching space. Situated away from the main campground road, section D provides plenty of peace and quiet. A short walk from section D is evidence of the last ice age. Glacial grooves

> *A day spent walking among Lake Erie's amazing natural resources is one long remembered.*

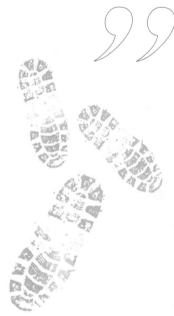

RATINGS

Beauty: ✰ ✰
Privacy: ✰ ✰
Spaciousness: ✰ ✰
Quiet: ✰ ✰
Security: ✰ ✰ ✰
Cleanliness: ✰ ✰ ✰

ADDRESS:	1169 N. Buck Road Lakeside-Marble-head, OH 43440-9610
OPERATED BY:	ODNR Division of State Parks
INFORMATION:	(419) 734-5857; www.dnr.state .oh.us/parks
RESERVATIONS:	(866) 644-6727; www.ohio.reserve world.com
OPEN:	Year-round; limited facilities in winter
SITES:	189 nonelectric; 351 electric
EACH SITE:	Picnic table, fire ring
ASSIGNMENT:	Reservable sites; walk-in sites first come, first served
REGISTRATION:	At entrance station; check in 3 p.m., check out 1 p.m.
FACILITIES:	Showers, flush toilets, laundry, camp store, game room, boat launch ramp, fish-cleaning station, bike rentals, disc golf, swimming beach
PARKING:	At each site
FEE:	$22 nonelectric; $27 electric
ELEVATION:	586 feet
RESTRICTIONS:	*Pets:* Permitted in sections D and G on leash, not permitted in section A *Fires:* In fire ring *Alcohol:* Prohibited *Vehicles:* 2 per site *Other:* Limit 6 persons per site; quiet hours 10 p.m.–6 a.m.; gathering firewood prohibited

were left behind in exposed rock by the glaciers' last retreat. The grooves are open for campers to walk on and touch.

The harbors are protected from Lake Erie's waves, offering calm waters for kayaking. Add a camera to the paddling adventure and chances are high you will find plenty of waterfowl to photograph. The rocks protecting the harbor shoreline host a variety of wild things for viewing or photographing. Snakes are plentiful and regularly expose themselves on the rocks before or after feeding on baitfish and frogs. During the three primary camping seasons, East Harbor State Park hosts several conservational programs for campers to participate in, some of which provide an in-depth look into the wildlife that thrives there. East Harbor State Park is a boater's ideal base camp. A large parking area near the registration station provides tent campers with a place to park their boat trailers overnight. East Harbor's hiking trails lead campers through the lakeshore's diverse habitats. It's wise to take along a bird identification guidebook on your hike, as hundreds of species visit the area. Some live here year-round, while others are merely resting as they journey through.

This region of Lake Erie is rich with sightseeing opportunities. A historic lighthouse at the tip of Marble-head Peninsula is skirted by a rocky shoreline. The waves continue to work on those rocks, exhibiting a great show of nature's power. Several wineries squeeze some of the finest wine-making grapes in the world, which grow well in the rich soil and are caressed by Lake Erie's breezes. Back at the state park, a 1,500-foot sand beach awaits swimmers. Looking out from Lake Erie's shore, islands appear on the horizon. A ferry system carries visitors to those islands daily. For information on ferry schedules and rates, visit **www.portclinton.org/ferryboats.**

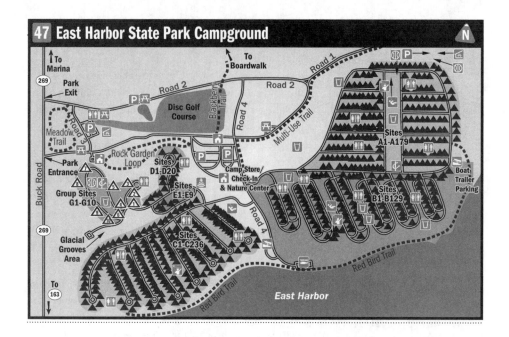

47 East Harbor State Park Campground

N

To Marina

269 Park Exit

Road 2

To Boardwalk

Road 2

Road 1

Disc Golf Course

Blackberry Trail

Road 4

Multi-Use Trail

Sites A1–A179

Meadow Trail

Road 3

Park Entrance

Rock Garden Loop

Sites D1–D20

Camp Store/ Check-In & Nature Center

Sites E1–E9

Group Sites G1–G10

Sites B1–B129

Boat Trailer Parking

269

Glacial Grooves Area

Sites C1–C236

Road 4

Red Bird Trail

Red Bird Trail

Buck Road

To 163

East Harbor

GETTING THERE

From OH 2 on the north shore of Sandusky Bay, take OH 269 north 2.3 miles to OH 163. Go east on OH 163 for 0.4 mile to OH 269 north on the left. Travel 1 mile to the campground entrance on the right.

GPS COORDINATES

N41°32.689'
W82°49.226'

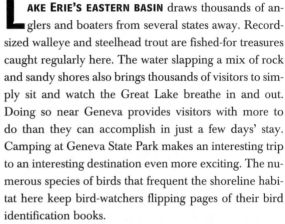

48
GENEVA
STATE PARK

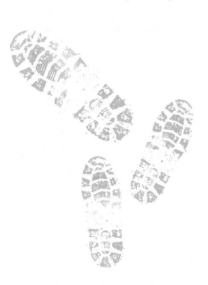

> *This summertime resort offers both manmade fun and natural attractions.*

LAKE ERIE'S EASTERN BASIN draws thousands of anglers and boaters from several states away. Record-sized walleye and steelhead trout are fished-for treasures caught regularly here. The water slapping a mix of rock and sandy shores also brings thousands of visitors to simply sit and watch the Great Lake breathe in and out. Doing so near Geneva provides visitors with more to do than they can accomplish in just a few days' stay. Camping at Geneva State Park makes an interesting trip to an interesting destination even more exciting. The numerous species of birds that frequent the shoreline habitat here keep bird-watchers flipping pages of their bird identification books.

A 2-mile paved path runs from the camp entrance to the summer resort town of Geneva-On-The-Lake, east of the park. Both bikers and walkers share the trail. This summer hotspot offers waterslides, arcades, and other beach-town entertainment. The climate and soil of this region are conducive to growing grapes, and dozens of vineyards dot the area. A glass of locally made wine with a few fresh walleye fillets make a dandy camp dinner.

Tucked back in a woodlot, 700 feet from the Lake Erie shore, is Geneva State Park's campground. Most campers that stay at this campground are either boating or fishing Lake Erie, or enjoying some other Great Lakes–region activity. A swimming beach is only a quarter-mile walk from the campground entrance. Camping families wanting a touch of beach vacation can quench their thirst by putting a foot in Lake Erie's cool, refreshing water. Past the gate at the campground office, overflow camping is offered in the form of seven sites on an open lawn. This is not the most aesthetically pleasing spot to pitch a tent, but during the busy boating season running from spring through early fall, the spots come in handy. If you do bring your boat, a six-lane boat ramp at the marina sits just outside the

RATINGS

Beauty: ✿ ✿
Privacy: ✿ ✿
Spaciousness: ✿ ✿
Quiet: ✿ ✿
Security: ✿ ✿ ✿
Cleanliness: ✿ ✿ ✿

campground. Concessions at the marina offer bait and boating supplies.

Sites 1–37 complete a circle that is popular with RVers during the summer season. Small trees are interspersed sparsely in this loop, offering little shade from the summer sun. Tent campers are better suited to sites 38 and 40 back on the main campground road and south of the 1–37 section. (Those two sites sit at the beginning of the campground's second section.) Sites 38 and 40 are well spaced and offer some privacy. The campground contour is nearly flat, which means that on rainy days, water pools at several of the sites in the 38–93 loop.

A spur off the 38–93 loop has sites that sit a couple feet higher than the wetlands surrounding the campground. This drier branch is also void of any pet droppings, as pets are not permitted in this area. At the end of this branch is site 68, which drains well, even with ample shade. The insects come out at night along the big lake's brushy flora, so be prepared to fend off mosquitoes. The vegetation near the beach area includes a few species that are rare in Ohio, such as the beach pea and sea rockets—Atlantic coast natives.

Note: Juvenile campers must provide written permission from parents or guardians to camp alone.

KEY INFORMATION

ADDRESS:	4499 Padanarum Road Geneva, OH 44041
OPERATED BY:	ODNR Division of State Parks
INFORMATION:	(440) 466-5069; www.dnr.state.oh.us/parks
RESERVATIONS:	(866) 644-6727; www.ohio.reserveworld.com
OPEN:	Year-round, but showers and store closed November–April
SITES:	89 electric; 7 nonelectric
EACH SITE:	Picnic table, fire ring
ASSIGNMENT:	Reservable sites; walk-in sites first come, first served
REGISTRATION:	If office closed, self register
FACILITIES:	Showers, flush toilets, laundry, store, boat launch, fish-cleaning station, swimming beach
PARKING:	At each site; overflow parking in north visitor's lot
FEE:	$29 electric; $21 nonelectric; $1 off Sun.–Thurs.; $2 off in winter
ELEVATION:	582 feet
RESTRICTIONS:	*Pets:* On leash at least 6 feet in length; no pets at sites 53–69 *Fires:* In fire ring *Alcohol:* Prohibited *Vehicles:* 2 per site *Other:* Quiet hours 10 p.m.–6 a.m.; gathering firewood prohibited; limit 6 persons per site

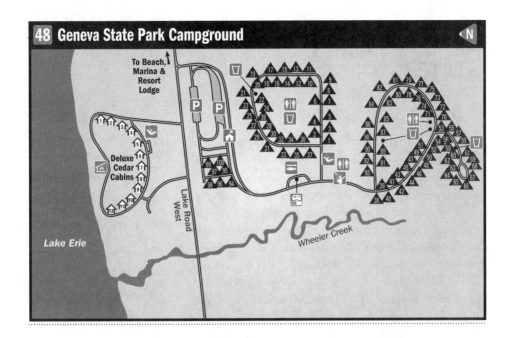

GETTING THERE

From I-90 Exit 218, south of Geneva, take OH 534 north 5.43 miles to the park entrance on the left. Follow the park road for 1.88 miles to the campground entrance on the left.

GPS COORDINATES

N41°51.248'
W80°59.146'

49
KELLEYS ISLAND STATE PARK

KELLEYS ISLAND is the most pleasant, quiet, and naturally blessed land mass in Lake Erie. The island hosts the North Pond Nature Preserve adjoining the campground's south boundary, a 30-acre sanctuary accessible by a boardwalk, hiking trail, and viewing tower. The star natural attractions of Kelleys Island are the Glacial Grooves left from the latest ice age. The grooves are impressive: 430 feet long, 15 feet deep, and 35 feet wide. Visitors have access to view all sides of the glacier's footprint with a surrounding walkway with several interpretative stations along the self-guided tour. Angling is a popular activity on and around the island. Campers have access to public fishing, and many fishing charters offer their services to visitors wanting to catch a few of the infamous Lake Erie Walleye. The Kelleys Island Ferry Boat Line is located in Marblehead and provides year-round service, weather permitting; call (419) 798-9763 for more information.

When considering camping on an island, it's amusing to think of Robinson Crusoe's story of island survival. Camping on Kelleys Island, however, brings much more pleasant thoughts after walking the gravel shoreline and inspecting the ancient stones, then pondering their story, which took place over thousands of years. The campground offers amenities that Robinson would have appreciated. Sitting several yards from and higher than the lake's edge are ten tent-only sites apart from the main campground circuit. Take a left after passing the campground office to find the short, horseshoe-shaped lane accessing those sites.

The first four sites are void of trees, which are missed after playing under the sun all day. The remainder of the tent-only section is interlaced in a young woodlot. Sites 117 and 119 are outside the horseshoe but are close to Division Street. During the summer vacation season, the regular buzz of golf carts scooting up and down the street

> *The glacial grooves are a must-see, as there is no other display like them in the world.*

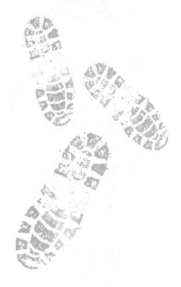

RATINGS

Beauty: ☆ ☆ ☆
Privacy: ☆ ☆
Spaciousness: ☆ ☆
Quiet: ☆ ☆
Security: ☆ ☆ ☆
Cleanliness: ☆ ☆ ☆

ADDRESS:	920 Division Street Kelleys Island, OH 43438
OPERATED BY:	ODNR Division of State Parks
INFORMATION:	(419) 746-2546; www.dnr.state .oh.us/parks
RESERVATIONS:	(866) 644-6727; www.ohio.reserve world.com
OPEN:	April–October
SITES:	45 nonelectric; 82 electric
EACH SITE:	Picnic table, fire ring
ASSIGNMENT:	Reservable sites; walk-in sites first come, first served
REGISTRATION:	Self-registration station at camp- ground office, if office closed
FACILITIES:	Showers, flush toilets, camp store, game room, boat launch ramp, fish- cleaning station, swimming beach
PARKING:	At each site
FEE:	$30 lakefront; $25 nonelectric
ELEVATION:	592 feet
RESTRICTIONS:	*Pets:* On leash only *Fires:* In fire ring *Alcohol:* Prohibited *Vehicles:* 1 per site *Other:* No mopeds or golf carts in campground; quiet hours 10 p.m.–8 a.m.; gathering firewood prohibit- ed; limit 6 persons per site; limit 2 tents per site; 14- day stay maximum

will disturb that nap you hoped to take. The horseshoe turn is skirted by sites 121 and 122, which are Rent-A-Camps. These include a high-wall tent, camp stove, cots and sleeping pads, lantern, cooler, fire ring, and picnic table with canopy as a package to rent. Sites 124 and 127 are the following two sites on the lane, and they are is-land yurts—round-sided, wood-frame structures covered with canvas and situated on a wooden deck serving as the floor. Those rentals occupy the best four sites in the campground for tent camping, and they come with a view of the beach. Site 128 is the last site on the lane that sits between the lane and Lake Erie. It's a long site, near-ly 20 yards from the parking pad to the water's edge, and is decorated with three-foot limestone boulders for erosion control—they also provide crevices for hiding harmless water snakes.

Neighboring the tent-only sites section and on the waterfront are sites 101, 103, and 104. They are the second-best sites for tent camping with two rows of trees growing a couple yards from the bouldered shoreline, but paralleling the shore. Parked in a folding camping chair at site 103 at daybreak, a camper will be treated to a sunrise show only found on an island. Site 101 sits next to a rentable picnic shelter and site 97 is on the other side. Across the lane is site 94, not a waterfront site but with a view of a waterfront site, and the main shower house is only a few yards away. After site 97, there are seven more waterfront sites before reaching the lane's turn inland and to the heart of the campground. The last waterfront site is 85, and next to it is a lane that leads to a fish-cleaning shed that is open to all campers.

The campground's interior sites are split into three groups. Sites 1–34 are laid out along both sides of a branch paralleling Division Street, with only a sparse row of trees situated between the road and the sites. A shorter branch between that lane and Lake Erie, but similar in shape, holds sites 35–58. All of the sites on those two branches offer lawn camping, with some stray shade from the occasional tree. Sites 59–71 line a lane between the two branches and the lake and are a bit more isolated.

To the northwest of the campground is another state nature preserve, the North Shore Alvar. Alvars

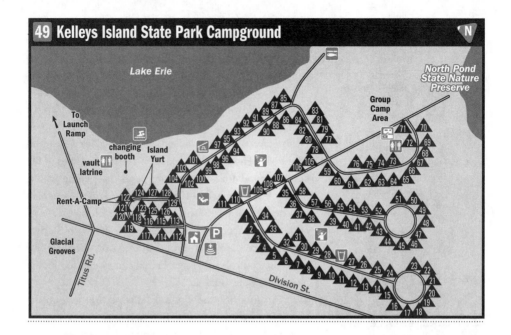

are horizontal stripes of limestone exposed by glaciers and kept in view by environmental forces such as the wind and waves working over Kelleys Island's north shoreline. The formations support rare and endangered species of plants such as the northern bog violet. To experience this special place, go past the Glacial Grooves State Memorial until the road dead-ends at the boaters' parking area. Enter the preserve on the state park trail to the northwest.

GETTING THERE

From Marblehead, board the Kelleys Island Ferry from 510 West Main Street. From the ferry dock on the southern point of Kelleys Island, follow East Lake Shore Road 0.26 mile to Division Street on the right. Follow Division Street 1.44 miles to the campground entrance on the right.

GPS COORDINATES

N41°36.874'
W82°42.385'

SOUTH BASS ISLAND STATE PARK

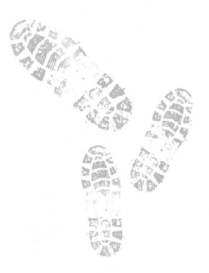

> *Cliff-top campsites provide gorgeous views of Lake Erie.*

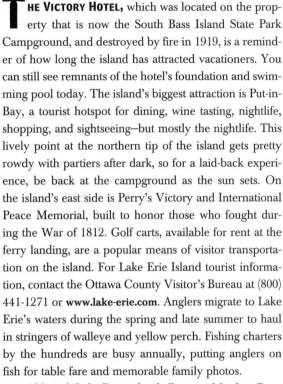

THE VICTORY HOTEL, which was located on the property that is now the South Bass Island State Park Campground, and destroyed by fire in 1919, is a reminder of how long the island has attracted vacationers. You can still see remnants of the hotel's foundation and swimming pool today. The island's biggest attraction is Put-in-Bay, a tourist hotspot for dining, wine tasting, nightlife, shopping, and sightseeing—but mostly the nightlife. This lively point at the northern tip of the island gets pretty rowdy with partiers after dark, so for a laid-back experience, be back at the campground as the sun sets. On the island's east side is Perry's Victory and International Peace Memorial, built to honor those who fought during the War of 1812. Golf carts, available for rent at the ferry landing, are a popular means of visitor transportation on the island. For Lake Erie Island tourist information, contact the Ottawa County Visitor's Bureau at (800) 441-1271 or **www.lake-erie.com**. Anglers migrate to Lake Erie's waters during the spring and late summer to haul in stringers of walleye and yellow perch. Fishing charters by the hundreds are busy annually, putting anglers on fish for table fare and memorable family photos.

Although Lake Erie is the shallowest of the five Great Lakes, its beauty runs deep, and there is no better observation point than atop a stone cliff at South Bass Island campground. Even while registering at the campground office, views of the lake will capture your attention. Because the campground is located on the windward side of South Bass Island, the waves are taller here. After you force yourself to get back in your vehicle and head up into the shaded campground, sites 130–135 are on the left, at the edge of the stone cliff that gradually gains elevation. The six sites also overlook a stony beach to the south and a busy boat ramp and concessions that rent jet skis in the summer. The sites are well spaced but, be aware, sit on a slope toward the cliff edge that has no safety fence.

RATINGS

Beauty: ✿ ✿ ✿ ✿
Privacy: ✿ ✿
Spaciousness: ✿ ✿
Quiet: ✿ ✿
Security: ✿ ✿ ✿
Cleanliness: ✿ ✿ ✿

LAKE ERIE REGION

The campground's paved lane splits after site 130; there is no choice but to go right on this one-way route. The narrow lane ramps up to a flat hilltop covered with a tight tree canopy made up of a mix of mature hardwood trees. Sites 1–70 cover the hilltop, sitting close together, with only a few feet between each. This is where the RVs gather, and the view of Lake Erie is blocked by treetops growing along the cliff section. The sites featuring great lake views and breezes are reserved for tent campers only. The one-way lane will pass site 14 on the left, go straight to a "T" in the road, and go left. Sites 75–77 and sites 87–94 sit on the right and offer a tent spot on a hump in the woods, just a few steps from the parking pad. Across from site 87 are sites 78–86, sitting around the outside of a loop that drops down, away from the main campground lane.

Sites 95–101 are at the highest point on the lake cliff, and parking for those sites is in a shared parking area on the right side of the lane as the lane makes a turn and faces downhill toward the campground entrance. Site 101 is the northernmost site and the most private. Each site is allowed 10 square yards of campsite. The lane continues south to the remaining lakeview sites. Sites 102–109 are set closer to the lane than to the cliff edge but still offer amazing views of the lake. The next small parking area on the right is for sites 112–117, which are shoved out toward the edge of the rock face. A shower house is centrally located among the cliffside sites next to this parking area. If small children are part of the Lake Erie island campout, consider sites 106, 110, 119, or 120, as they do provide decent views of the sunset but are on the opposite side of the campground lane, a safe distance from the cliff. Thirty yards from returning to the one-way split near the lane's beginning, a fish cleaning shed is available near site 122. Site 125 sits on a knoll, a grandstand of a site for the great Lake Erie "show."

KEY INFORMATION

ADDRESS:	1523 Catawba Ave. Put-in-Bay, OH 43456
OPERATED BY:	ODNR Division of State Parks
INFORMATION:	(419) 734-4425; www.dnr.state .oh.us/parks
RESERVATIONS:	(866) 644-6727; www.ohio.reserve world.com
OPEN:	April–October
SITES:	120 nonelectric
EACH SITE:	Picnic table, fire ring
ASSIGNMENT:	Reservable sites; walk-in sites first come, first served
REGISTRATION:	Self-registration station at campground office, if office closed
FACILITIES:	Showers, flush toilets, camp store, game room, boat launch ramp, fish-cleaning station, swimming beach
PARKING:	At each site
FEE:	$28
ELEVATION:	590 feet
RESTRICTIONS:	*Pets:* On leash only *Fires:* In fire ring *Alcohol:* Prohibited *Vehicles:* 1 per site *Other:* No mopeds or golf carts in campground; quiet hours 10 p.m.–8 a.m.; gathering firewood prohibited; limit 6 persons per site

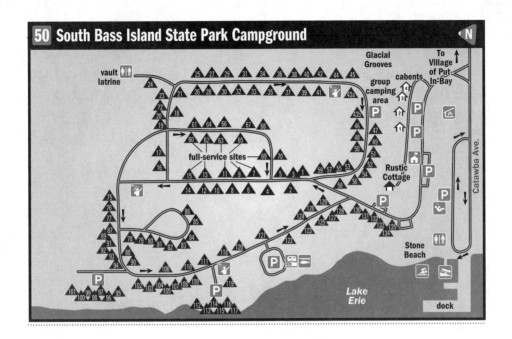

50 South Bass Island State Park Campground

GETTING THERE

From the northernmost point on Catawba Island, take the ferry (**www.millers ferry.com** or (800) 500-2421) north 3 miles to South Bass Island. Follow Langram Road northeast 0.98 mile to Meechen Road on the left. Travel 0.43 mile northwest to Catawba Road and turn left. The park entrance is down the hill on the right.

GPS COORDINATES

N41°38.518'
W82°50.154'

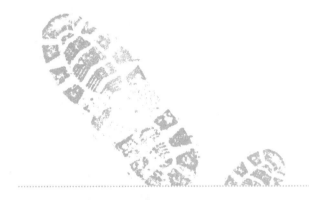

APPENDIXES & INDEX

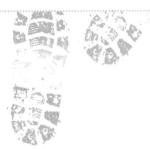

APPENDIX A: SOURCES OF INFORMATION

OHIO DEPARTMENT OF NATURAL RESOURCES (ODNR)
Division of Parks
2045 Morse Road, Building C
Columbus, OH 43229-6693
(614) 265-6561
www.dnr.state.oh.us/parks

ODNR DIVISION OF FORESTRY
2045 Morse Road, Building H
Columbus, OH 43229-6693
(877) 247-8733
www.ohiodnr.com/forestry

ODNR DIVISION OF NATURAL AREAS AND PRESERVES
2045 Morse Road, Building C
Columbus, OH 43229-6693
(614) 265-6453
www.ohiodnr.com/dnap

ODNR DIVISION OF WILDLIFE
2045 Morse Road, Building G
Columbus, OH 43229-6693
(800) WILDLIFE
www.wildohio.com

OHIO TOURISM DIVISION
P.O. Box 1001
Columbus, OH 43216-1001
(800) BUCKEYE
www.discoverohio.com

WAYNE NATIONAL FOREST
13700 US Highway 33
Nelsonville, OH 45764
(740) 753-0101
www.fs.usda.gov/wayne

U.S. ARMY CORPS OF ENGINEERS
36007 State Route 715
Warsaw, OH 43844-9534
(740) 824-4343
www.corpslakes.us

SANDUSKY COUNTY PARK DISTRICT
1970 Countryside Place
Fremont, OH 43420
(888) 200-5577
www.sanduskycountyparks.com

MUSKINGUM WATERSHED CONSERVANCY DISTRICT
1319 3rd Street NW; P.O. Box 349
New Philadelphia, OH 44663
(877) 363-8500
www.mwcd.org

FIVE RIVERS METROPARKS
1375 E. Siebenthaler Avenue
Dayton, OH 45414
(937) 275-PARK
www.metroparks.org

GEAUGA PARK DISTRICT
9160 Robinson Road
Chardon, OH 44024
(800) 536-4006
www.geaugaparkdistrict.org

HAMILTON COUNTY PARK DISTRICT
10245 Winton Road
Cincinnati, OH 45231
(513) 521-7275
www.greatparks.org

AMERICAN ELECTRIC POWER
1 Riverside Plaza
Columbus, OH 43215-2372
(614) 716-1000
**www.aep.com/environmental/
recreation/recland**

APPENDIX B: CAMPING EQUIPMENT CHECKLIST

The basic utensils and smaller items I routinely use on camping trips are conveniently packed in a large storage bin that transfers easily from garage to car in seconds. It makes preparing for a camping trip efficient. All I have to do is grab a tent and sleeping bag, gather food to bring, and away I go. If I donít have it when I get to my campsite, I figure I really didnít need it in the first place. Some of the basic items I do carry are:

COOKING UTENSILS
Biodegradable dish soap
Bottle opener/corkscrew
Coffee pot
Containers of salt, pepper, other favorite
    seasonings, cooking oil, sugar
Cups, dishes, bowls
Frying pan (cast iron)
Fuel for camp stove
Large water container
Lighter, matches, and so on
Pots with lids (at least two,
    large and medium)
Utensils, including big spoon, spatula,
    paring knife
Small camp stove
Tin foil

FIRST AID KIT
Antibiotic cream
Aspirin
Band-Aids, assorted sizes
Benadryl
Gauze pads
Insect repellent
Moleskin
Personal medications, clearly marked
Sunscreen/lip balm

SLEEPING GEAR
Pillow
Sleeping bag and liner (optional)
Sleeping pad (inflatable or insulated)
Tent with tub floor; tent fly, ground tarp

MISCELLANEOUS
Bath soap (biodegradable)
Camera and film
Camp chair
Candles
Cooler
Deck of cards
Duct tape
Fire starter
Flashlight or headlamp with fresh batteries
Foul-weather clothing
Paper towels
Plastic zip-top bags
Sunglasses
Toilet paper
Water bottle
Wool blanket

OPTIONAL
Barbecue grill
Binoculars (waterproof)
Field guides
Fishing gear
Lantern or tent candles
Maps, charts, other references and
    information

INDEX

DEAR CUSTOMERS AND FRIENDS,

SUPPORTING YOUR INTEREST IN OUTDOOR ADVENTURE, travel, and an active lifestyle is central to our operations, from the authors we choose to the locations we detail to the way we design our books. Menasha Ridge Press was incorporated in 1982 by a group of veteran outdoorsmen and professional outfitters. For many years now, we've specialized in creating books that benefit the outdoors enthusiast.

Almost immediately, Menasha Ridge Press earned a reputation for revolutionizing outdoors- and travel-guidebook publishing. For such activities as canoeing, kayaking, hiking, backpacking, and mountain biking, we established new standards of quality that transformed the whole genre, resulting in outdoor-recreation guides of great sophistication and solid content. Menasha Ridge continues to be outdoor publishing's greatest innovator.

The folks at Menasha Ridge Press are as at home on a white-water river or mountain trail as they are editing a manuscript. The books we build for you are the best they can be, because we're responding to your needs. Plus, we use and depend on them ourselves.

We look forward to seeing you on the river or the trail. If you'd like to contact us directly, join in at www.trekalong.com or visit us at www.menasharidge.com. We thank you for your interest in our books and the natural world around us all.

SAFE TRAVELS,

Bob Sehlinger

BOB SEHLINGER
PUBLISHER